Terry Tunnell
1988

12.69

The complete guide to cancer research!

CANCER

A COMPREHENSIVE TREATISE

Edited by **Frederick F. Becker**
University of Texas System Cancer Center
M. D. Anderson Hospital and Tumor Institute

The realization that cancer is a leading cause of death and disability throughout the world has prompted a vast amount of scientific research, with millions of dollars being invested in hope of finding a means of prevention or cure. With the publication of this much-needed work, specialists in this field have at their disposal a multivolume treatise of unparalleled breadth.

Leading authorities offer different points of view on important questions confronting cancer researchers and discuss past and present wide-scale research efforts. Examining the clinical foundations of the study of cancer, as well as its etiology and basic biology, this major systematic work should prove to be the fundamental scientific and medical guide for experimenters and clinicians.

D1218817

Cancer, Stress, and Death

SLOAN-KETTERING INSTITUTE CANCER SERIES

Series Editors:
ROBERT A. GOOD, Ph.D., M.D., and STACEY B. DAY, M.D., Ph.D., D.Sc.
Sloan-Kettering Institute for Cancer Research
New York, New York

GASTROINTESTINAL TRACT CANCER
Edited by Martin Lipkin, M.D., and Robert A. Good, Ph.D., M.D.

CANCER, STRESS, AND DEATH
Edited by Jean Taché, D. Sc., Hans Selye, C.C., M.D., Ph.D., D.Sc., and
Stacey B. Day, M.D., Ph.D., D.Sc.

Cancer, Stress, and Death

Edited by

Jean Taché, D. Sc.
International Institute of Stress
Pointe-Claire, Quebec, Canada

Hans Selye, C.C., M.D., Ph.D., D.Sc.
International Institute of Stress
Montreal, Quebec, Canada

and

Stacey B. Day, M.D., Ph.D., D.Sc.
Sloan-Kettering Institute for Cancer Research
New York, New York

PLENUM MEDICAL BOOK COMPANY
New York and London

Library of Congress Cataloging in Publication Data

Main entry under title:

Cancer, stress, and death.

(Sloan-Kettering Institute cancer series)
Bibliography: p.
Includes index.
1. Cancer — Psychosomatic aspects — Congresses. 2. Cancer — Psychological aspects — Congresses. 3. Stress (Physiology) — Congresses. 4. Stress (Psychology) — Congresses. 5. Death — Psychological aspects — Congresses. I. Taché, Jean. II. Selye, Hans, 1907-   III. Day, Stacey B. IV. Series: Sloan-Kettering Institute for Cancer Research, New York. Sloan-Kettering Institute cancer series.
RC261.A1C39   616.9'94'0019   78-27204
ISBN 0-306-40143-6

© 1979 Plenum Publishing Corporation
227 West 17th Street, New York, N.Y. 10011

Plenum Medical Book Company is an imprint of Plenum Publishing Corporation

Printed in the United States of America

And I would say
I am no doctor
I am a physician
I am your pilot
Come to guide your ship home to its last dock.

—From the "Last Dock" by Stacey B. Day

Participants

Pierre Band, M.D.
Director of Clinical Research
Montreal Cancer Institute
Montreal, Quebec H2L 4M1, Canada

Stephen Nye Barton, M.D., Ph.D.
Assistant Professor of Public Health
The University of Alabama in Birmingham
Birmingham, Alabama 35294
President, American Rural Health Association
Birmingham, Alabama 35205

Debbie Bowles, R.N., B.S.N., P.N.P.
St. Jude Children's Research Hospital
Memphis, Tennessee 38101

Aaron Bendich, Ph.D.
Member and Professor
Sloan-Kettering Institute for Cancer Research
New York, New York 10021

G.M. Brown, M.D., Ph.D.
Chairman, Department of Neurosciences
McMaster University
Hamilton, Ontario L8S 4J9, Canada

Eric J. Cassell, M.D., F.A.C.P.
Clinical Professor, Department of Public Health
The New York Hospital
Cornell University Medical College
New York, New York 10021

Barbara G. Cox, B.S.
Executive Editor and Manager
Biomedical Publications, Ross Laboratories
Columbus, Ohio 43216

Stacey B. Day, M.D., Ph.D., D.Sc.
Member and Professor
Sloan-Kettering Institute for Cancer Research
New York, New York 10021

Joel Elkes, M.D.
Distinguished Service Professor
Johns Hopkins University
Baltimore, Maryland 21218
Visiting Professor
McMaster University
Hamilton, Ontario L8S 4J9, Canada

Robert Fulton, Ph.D.
Professor of Sociology and Director
Center for Death Education and Research
University of Minnesota
Minneapolis, Minnesota 55455

Irwin H. Krakoff, M.D.
Professor and Director
Vermont Regional Cancer Center
University of Vermont
Burlington, Vermont 05401

Terence E. Lear, F.R.C.P.I., D.P.M., F.R.C.Psych.
Physician and Consultant Psychiatrist
St. Crispin Hospital
Northampton, England NN2 6JF

Martin G. Lewis, M.D., M.R.C.(Path.)
Chairman, Department of Pathology
Georgetown University School of Medicine and Dentistry
Washington D.C. 20007

Wolfgang Luthe, M.D.
Scientific Director, Oskar Vogt Institute
Visiting Professor
Kyūshū University
Fukuoka, Japan

Balfour Mount, M.D., F.R.C.S.(C)
Director, Palliative Care Unit
Royal Victoria Hospital
McGill University
Montreal, Quebec H3A 1A1, Canada

Janet Schyving Payne, A.C.S.W.
St. Jude Children's Research Hospital
Memphis, Tennessee 38101

Paul J. Rosch, A.B., M.A., M.D., F.A.C.P.
Chairman
American Institute of Stress
301 Park Avenue
New York, New York 10022

Milagros Salas, Ph.D.
Research Fellow
Montreal Cancer Institute
Montreal, Quebec H2L 4M1, Canada

Hans Selye, C.C., M.D., Ph.D., D.Sc.
President, International Institute of Stress
University of Montreal
Montreal, Quebec H3C 3J7, Canada

Jean Taché, D.Sc.
Director, Center for Applied Stress Studies
Pointe-Claire, Quebec H9S 4J7, Canada
President, The Stress Corporation
8100 Paseo del Ocaso
La Jolla, California 92037

Mary L. S. Vachon, R.N., M.A.
Community Resources Section
Clarke Institute of Psychiatry
Toronto, Ontario M5T 1R8, Canada

Edmund Yunis, M.D., Ph.D.
Professor of Pathology
Harvard Medical School and Chief, Division of Immunogenetics
Sidney Farber Cancer Institute
Boston, Massachusetts 02115

Foreword

When I delivered the keynote address at our joint 1977 symposium on Cancer, Stress, and Death in Montreal, I took great pride in announcing my unique qualification for this singular honor—I had survived a normally fatal cancer, a histiocytic reticulosarcoma that had developed under the skin of my thigh several years previously.

Faced with the physical and emotional realities of this situation, I refused to retreat from life in desperation. I immediately underwent surgery and cobalt therapy, but insisted on knowing my chances for a lasting recovery, which at that time seemed far from encouraging. Although I knew it would take tremendous self-discipline, I was determined to continue living and working without worrying about the outcome.

I suppressed any thoughts of my ostensibly imminent death, but rewrote my will, including in it several suggestions for the continuation of my work by my colleagues. Having taken care of that business, I promptly forced myself to disregard the whole calamity. I immersed myself in my work—and I survived! But, of course, this was not my only reason for my feelings of pride and accomplishment.

I have since succeeded in creating the International Institute of Stress, and one of its first major symposiums was specifically arranged to highlight the interrelation between stress, cancer, and death. The Memorial Sloan-Kettering Cancer Center added prestige to our venture by cosponsoring this event and ensuring the participation of many leading experts, whose work on stress and cancer is well represented in this volume.

We know very little about the possible relationship between stress and cancer, but no one can ever doubt that stress enters into every kind of human activity and that it is responsible for many of today's diseases of adaptation. Indeed, under general stress, it is always the weakest link in the chain—the weakest part of the human mechanism—that breaks down first. There is no reason, therefore, to exclude stress from being a critical factor in the development of cancer, which in itself is also a major source of stress in these patients. I think it would not be very difficult to understand that a person who is about to die of cancer is under stress, at least in the original sense of the word—what we now prefer to call *distress.*

Several years ago, I personally did an experiment which amused me very much. I implanted chemically inert pyrex rings of a certain shape under the skin of some rats, and they produced a sarcoma in 100% of these animals. I still do not know how this came about, but I suspect the pyrex rings must have been highly irritating. Rather surprisingly, broken pieces of pyrex failed to duplicate this effect. We had to use pyrex rings of specific dimensions because any other shape was ineffective. This provides clear-cut evidence that local stress (discussed in Chapter 2) is carcinogenic only under certain conditions.

So the possibilities seem limitless, especially when one considers the relationship between stress, altered emotional states, and cancer. Perhaps, as Paul Rosch of New York has suggested, cancer might even be an attempt by the human organism to regenerate tissues and organs and even limbs, as lower animals are able to do spontaneously. Going further, one might say that "the ultimate health of the organism, like that of society, appears to depend on how well or appropriately its constituent units communicate with one another." As I said in my book *Stress without Distress,* "the indispensability of this disciplined, orderly mutual cooperation is best illustrated by its opposite—the development of a cancer, whose most characteristic feature is that it cares only for itself."

I believe that new findings in cancer research will eventually provide many answers to mankind's everyday psychosocial problems. I do know that my own experience with the disease helped me to develop a very satisfactory code of conduct, and it is my hope that the various contributions to this book will take us a little further toward a more coherent theory on cancer, one that will correlate the vast multitude of findings in the scientific literature on stress, cancer, and death.

Hans Selye, C.C., M.D., Ph.D., D.Sc.
President, International Institute of Stress
University of Montreal
Montreal, Quebec, Canada

Preface

Oliver Wendell Holmes, speaking of the joy of life, remarked of Malebranche that if God held in one hand truth and in the other the pursuit of truth, the grand gentleman would say, "Lord, the truth is for Thee alone; give me the pursuit." It is the *pursuit* to its ulterior spiritual end—to death—that most thinking people, I believe, would turn, and it is to this end that the integrated views in this book are directed.

The ideas and concepts presented here originated with colleagues in intellectually diverse disciplines. The matters of which they speak and the research which they relate bridge a variety of fields of learning and should contribute to a broader and more sensitive understanding of cancer, stress, and death. Their ideas permit an elucidation and analysis of the consequences of those fields and of the different multicentric cultures that make up our rapidly shrinking world.

If we are not able to master the induction and process of ideas in these fields precisely (for the dimensions are too wide), our efforts at integration of interdisciplinary learning are at least beginning. There is more and more interest in and felicity for work in the *nonworld* of spaces that have existed between disciplines. Slowly such nonworld spaces, through the efforts of those few who are laboring in between disciplines, are closing. Note is being taken of their efforts to synthesize professional knowledge of what has been virtually left as a serious gap in the backdrop of our learning. This book presents evidence rather than testimony to those results pioneered in new dimensions of both contributory and participatory education.

Interest generated by this colloquium should therefore emphasize discussions and ideas from papers contributed by those who have labored at what might appropriately be called the grassroots level of the intellectual constructs of our society. Here, bridging gaps, cementing disciplines, and forging communions from these nonworlds, many talents have formed the concepts that are increasingly regarded as *interdisciplinary communications and learning*. These constructs, which are secured from the spaces of the nonworlds, form the new matrices of contemporary advances in scholarship and education.

Out of this testing work has come the thought-provoking areas of biosocial development, the sociological aspects of medicine inherent in such viewpoints as the patient-as-a-person, an understanding of interacting cultures, including science (for science is very much a culture), and important new syntheses and visions many of which are intrinsic in the observations on cancer, stress, and death presented here.

The Montreal colloquium was of value in encouraging and setting forth Malebranche's pursuit of truth in the will of the integrated philosophy just described. Perhaps Oliver Wendell Holmes himself might approve of the convening of tasks evident in studies of psychophysiology of stress, concepts of the brain as a self-regulating organ, the value and need of death education, and fascinating strengths beyond prospect, of cultural anthropology as an analytical instrument for evaluation of cultural transformations, sociological problems, and paradoxes and apparent incoherencies in the diversity of cultures within which all must live, and to which all must respond. Wise utilization and keen interpretation, using interdisciplinary analysis reasonably, promise a more sensitive appreciation of life forces that beget so many of our shared problems, including those of cancer, stress, and death.

This volume, and the themes it evokes, evolved from a cooperative, international, interdisciplinary, educational exchange that met under the sponsorship of the Sloan-Kettering Institute for Cancer Research (Biosciences Communication and Education), and the institute directed by Hans Selye, devoted to the research and elucidation of stress—the International Institute of Stress in Montreal, Canada.

It is by such socially oriented health research programs that more accessible, more profoundly human, and more participatory public attention can be brought to bear in fields of health education that benefit society, and that are of critical concern to patients as well as to physicians.

Stacey B. Day

Contents

Stress as a Cause of Disease

Jean Taché, D.Sc.

In developing the concept of stress, the attention of the researcher was focused on the response of the individual to stimuli: How does the body deal with demands arising from the environment? What reactions develop? How is equilibrium restored? Each problem arises in the individual, and successful coping activities are measured by his capacity to maintain or restore homeostasis. The stimuli themselves seem of interest only inasmuch as they can elicit a common response.

Once we have made the point of a general response to demands from the environment, we must analyze the mechanisms through which this response is mediated; then the nature of the stimuli takes on a new importance. The existence of a so-called first mediator (or first mediators) has been postulated in order to bridge the gap between the perception of the stressor and the common initiating of a response. Obviously there is a missing link—one which will explain how demands, whatever their nature, are transcribed into language understood by the cells in which the common response is initiated. Furthermore, the stimuli are also of interest

Jean Taché • Director, Center for Applied Stress Studies, Pointe-Claire, Quebec H9S 4J7, Canada. President, The Stress Corporation, 8100 Paseo del Ocaso, La Jolla, California 92037.

1

because interactions between specific and nonspecific aspects of the responses are possible; and in the final analysis, stressors may be a cause of—or a factor in—the development of a number of diseases, via many of the hormonal modifications they induce.

The Concept of Stress

The concept of stress was first formulated by Hans Selye in 1936.[1] Since then, the original definition has been honed to greater precision. Distinctions have been made (e.g., differentiating between *stress* and *stressor*) and oversights have been corrected (e.g., the mistaken conclusion that only noxious agents could induce stress).[2,3] Without delving into details, [4] we would like to describe the present status of the stress concept, indicating various points that are necessary to the understanding of how stress can be seen as a cause of disease.

Stress, "the nonspecific response of the body to any demand," is a process of adaptation which develops as a reaction to a stimulus (called the *stressor*) and is manifested through changes in hormone levels and in the size of many organs.

Stress is *nonspecific* in its causation: it is a general response elicited by psychological, physical, or chemical agents. Most stimuli elicit very characteristic responses by which they can be recognized; these responses are known as specific effects. The subcutaneous injection of an irritant will cause inflammation in that area; when a person is hot, he will sweat and lose some of his excess body heat; when he is cold, he will shiver, and through rapid muscle contraction, heat will be generated; during a game of tennis or a sprint around a race track, pulse rate and pulmonary respiration increase substantially as more blood flows to the muscles with the needed oxygen. However, at the same time that these specific reactions occur, a nonspecific effect—i.e., one that is common to all stressors—can be observed in the form of stereotyped modifications. The morphological and biochemical aspects of this response have been well documented,[5] but the psychological effect or behavioral aspects should not be overlooked.[6] It is this general—not *agent-specific*—reaction that is stress.

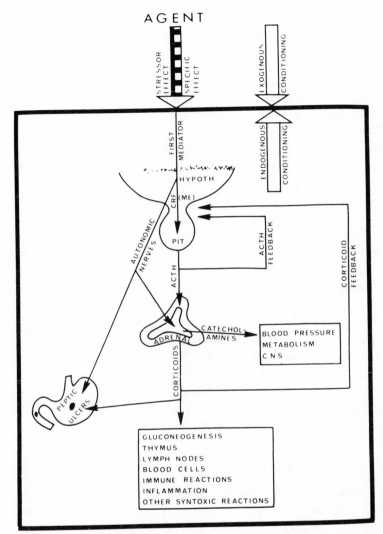

AGENT

Figure 1. Stereotyped response to various stimuli. Any demand on our body will determine a specific response by which it can usually be identified. It also elicits a stereotyped response characteristic of stress, as summarized in this diagram. The large dark frame represents an individual; the reactions indicated refer to the main pathway of adaptation in higher vertebrates and man. Sometimes, the specific effect on an agent will interact with some phase of this stereotyped response and modify it so that it no longer seems general. The response to a stressor is not exactly the same in all individuals: this is due to the fact that each individual is unique because of his conditioning factors—which, to a great extent, determine his sensitivity and the area of reaction.

Stereotyped Modifications

Readily observable, common morphological changes follow exposure to stressors: the adrenals in animals submitted to severe stress procedures become darker, and over the course of a few days increase in size; the thymus involutes; and gastric ulcers develop. This triad of morphological symptoms is not an exhaustive list of all the nonspecific changes in the body; there are other physical alterations that are not as apparent to the naked eye as those of the triad but which are characteristic of stress—as, for instance, changes in the weight of the gonads.

The body usually reacts to a stressor by the secretion of corticotropin-releasing factor (CRF) by cells in the area of the median eminence of the hypothalamus (Figure 1). CRF travels down the portal-venous system into the adenohypophysis, where it releases adrenocorticotropic hormone (ACTH). Carried by way of the vascular system, ACTH acts directly on the cortex of the adrenals, where it regulates the secretion of corticoids. These hormones induce a number of systemic modifications: gluconeogenesis is promoted at the expense of lipid reserves and even, if necessary, structure proteins; the thymus and lymph nodes involute; immune and inflammatory reactions decrease; and eosinopenia becomes evident. Simultaneously, through stimulation of the sympathetic nervous system, gastric or duodenal ulcers develop.

The General Adaptation Syndrome

It has been demonstrated time and time again that the manifestations of stress in laboratory animals evolve in at least three stages, which together constitute the general adaptation syndrome (G.A.S.) (Figure 2). When a stressor is first applied, an *alarm reaction* develops, during which resistance falls below normal and some hormones are secreted more abundantly. If the animal can outlive this initial phase and its defensive mechanisms can be put into action effectively, the level of resistance will rise and remain above normal for some time, depending upon the intensity of the stressor agent. Eventually, though, this *stage of resistance* will come to an end, as the animal can no longer maintain such a heightened

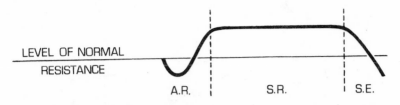

LEVEL OF NORMAL
RESISTANCE

A.R.   S.R.   S.E.

Figure 2. General adaptation syndrome: Resistance as modified during stress. The alarm reaction (A.R.) develops as a response to a stressor and resistance falls below normal; it rises considerably during the second phase, the stage of resistance (S.R.); eventually, the stage of exhaustion (S.E.) is reached when resistance drops dramatically and many diseases become apparent.

level of preparedness in response to the stimulus. The *stage of exhaustion*—the final phase of the G.A.S.—will ensue; diseases may become manifest and the animal may die sooner than normally happens under standard laboratory conditions.

Man and the G.A.S. The "call to arms" of the alarm reaction is triggered quite frequently in our bodies in response to daily events. If exposure to the stressor is short-lived, these modifications do not last and stress hormone levels rapidly revert to normal. However, if the stressor is intense or applied for a sufficiently long period, a form of adaptation will be reached during which stress hormone levels (e.g., ACTH, corticoids) remain elevated. But this adaptation is at a price. Although the teleologic significance of a modification is not easy to assess, one is forced to conclude from the series of modifications observed during stress that mobilization of the hypothalamus–hypophysis–adrenal axis leads to an increase in the capacity of the organism to be physically active, at the same time that other functions are decreased. This is indicated in morphological studies in a number of species of laboratory animals, for instance by the involution of the thymicolymphatic system and of the gonads, or by the decreased inflammatory response. Biochemically, a shift in secretion of adenohypophyseal hormones is also observed,[7] during which plasma levels of FSH, LH, prolactin, and growth hormone are significantly decreased (Figure 3) at the same time that ACTH (here represented by levels of corticosterone) is increased. Generally stated, this implies that the system necessary for immediate survival seems to take prece-

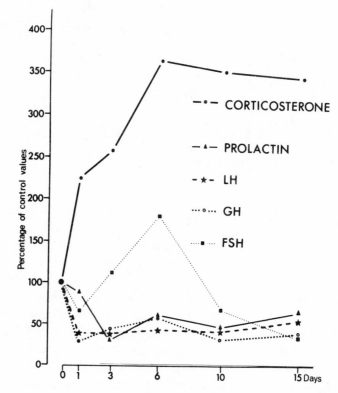

Figure 3. Effect of chronic immobilization (8 hours daily during 1, 3, 6, 10, or 15 days) on the plasma levels of some pituitary-related hormones in female rats: corticosterone, prolactin, luteinizing hormone (LH), growth hormone (GH), and follicle-stimulating hormone (FSH).

dence over secondary functions or lines of defense, such as reproduction or fight against inflammation, foreign proteins, etc.

A Stereotyped Yet Unique Response

Quite a few misunderstandings about the nature of stress arise from the fact that all people do not react to stressors equally or in exactly the same way. This should not be surprising, since there are no two identical individuals: each of us is conditioned by *endogenous* factors, i.e., genetically inherited traits such as familial diseases, proneness to certain maladies and weaknesses of specific organs, and *exogenous* factors, which include not only various physical conditions but also social, intellectual, and psychological elements which characterize the environment in which stressful events are experienced. These endogenous and exogenous factors combine to make each individual different from the next; and the stereotyped response, thus modulated, is unique for each person.

Measuring Stress

Obviously, stress is a complex phenomenon, and any one parameter utilized to measure it may well fall short of giving a realistic picture of the entire reaction. Under normal conditions, levels of ACTH and/or corticoids in the plasma or urine are considered to reflect the nonspecific adaptation process in the body; but, while stress can be monitored through biochemical tests, it should not be equated with secretion of ACTH, of corticoids, or of any other substance. The generalization made in the 1930's was not that diverse agents modify the weights of a number of organs (or the levels of certain hormones) but that the body reacts nonspecifically to diverse agents, of which the above-mentioned parameters are considered to be manifestations. One of the main interests of our Institute is to develop a valid stress test to be used for screening of individuals or of populations; such a test would lead to identification and counseling of susceptible individuals long before stress-related diseases become manifest.

Pluricausal Diseases

Diseases of adaptation are generally considered to be pluri-causal. Cardiovascular diseases—such as myocardial infarction and hypertension, two of the paramount killers in our age—are known to be associated to stress, which ranks with smoking, overweight, and lack of physical exercise as a prime risk factor. The role of stress in these diseases is described by some as being that of a permissive factor and by others as that of a triggering agent. The association, in any case, is so well documented that at the 1973 annual meeting of the Academy of Psychosomatic Medicine, a resolution read "Psychosocial stresses must be included among the recognized high-risk factors in myocardial infarction. . . . The psychiatrist and psychosocial team must be formally incorporated as an integral part of the Coronary Care Unit for every patient."

Coping Effectively with Situations

Although there is a biological given over which man has little or no control, there are a number of reactions which are learned and can be considered under his control to some degree. The relative importance of events to the individual is often a consequence of education, using the term in its broad sense. That man's brain can analyze any event in daily life in terms of survival certainly has not been without benefit to our species: the stereotyped response thus elicited has given him a tremendous advantage in his struggle for survival. In modern society, however, more and more decisions must be made which have no bearing on physical survival. That we are still conditioned to respond to everyday stressors in the age-old prehistoric way, in terms of survival, and that the mechanisms controlling physical activity are aroused to cope with problems which should be solved by the intellect, has become a biological anomaly.

One can perceive the situation in the following terms: In each one of us lies dormant a primeval man who in certain situations is aroused and imperiously takes command of the personality. Given the ancient problem-solving options available to him—fight or flight, both requiring physical activity—he can hardly come up with satisfactory solutions to modern problems, for they require reflection, negotiation, and compromise.

When one is taught to rely on this alarm reaction to deal with any stressor arising from the modern environment, the state of preparedness—which should be a transient one—sets in and develops into a habit, a way of life. The nervous and hormonal modifications through which the state of combat is attained are accompanied by other morphological and functional alterations at other levels. The longer-lasting this state, the more interactions and maladjustments are to be feared.

One has but to consider that emotional or psychogenic stress may induce modifications in the basal metabolic rate, [9] in vasopressin secretion,[10] in glucagon, serotonin, histamine, renin, angiotensin, and acetylcholine levels, and increases in plasma cholesterol, FFA, triglycerides, and lipoproteins, in addition to the well-known variations in levels of catecholamines and in adenohypophyseal and corticoid hormones.[11] All these modifications—if maintained for inordinate amounts of time—will lay the ground work for the development of disease.

Any perception the body analyzes as a threat to its survival will arouse the primordial man in us. And one cannot but decry the use and abuse of this ancient blind mechanism to exact a better or longer performance from other human beings. In a society starting to develop a worldwide consciousness of its oneness, these old mechanisms for survival should be considered precisely that, *old*, and as far as possible put to rest as new ones are developed to cope with stress in modern life. If the individual has learned to deal effectively with situations and events, he can arrive at specific adequate solutions to most problems without fearing his survival is at stake. In a nutshell, it is not that the ancient way of doing things is not useful: it is that this biological vestige is mobilized too often in circumstances where it need not be, given the high price it exacts in terms of health and well-being.

References

1. Selye, H. A syndrome produced by diverse nocuous agents. *Nature (Lond.)* 138: 32, 1936.
2. Lazarus, R. S. Psychological stress and coping in adaptation and illness. *Int J Psychiat Med* 5: 321–333, 1975.
3. Mason, J. W. A historical view of the stress field. Parts I and II. *J Human Stress* 1 (1): 6–12; 1 (2): 22–36, 1975.
4. Taché, J., and Selye, H. On stress and coping mechanisms. In: *Stress and Anxiety*, Vol. 5 (C. D. Spielberger and I. G. Sarason, eds.) Washington D.C.: Hemisphere Publishing Corporation, 1978.
5. Selye, H. *The Stress of Life.* New York: McGraw-Hill, 2nd edition, 1975.
6. Rowland, N. E., and Antelman, S. M. Stress-induced hyperphagia and obesity in rats: A possible model for understanding human obesity. *Science* 191:310–312, 1976.
7. Taché, Y., Du Ruisseau, P., Taché, J., Selye, H., and Collu, R. Shift in adenohypophyseal activity during chronic intermittent immobilization of rats. *Neuroendocrinology* 22: 325–336, 1976.
8. Academy of Psychosomatic Medicine, 20th Annual Meeting, November 20, 1973, Williamsburg, Virginia.

9. Corson, S. A., Corson, E. O., Kilrilcuk, V., Hajek, J., and Hajkova, M. Individual differences in oxygen consumption under emotional stress. *Fed Proc* 28: 648, 1969.

10. Lutz, B., Koch, B., and Mialhe, C. Sécrétion de l'hormone antidiurétique au cours de différents types d' aggression chez le Rat. *J Physiol (Paris)* 61 (supp. 1): 149–150, 1969.

11. Selye, H. *Stress in Health and Disease.* London: Butterworth, 1976.

Stress, Cancer, and the Mind

Hans Selye, C.C., M.D., Ph.D., D.Sc.

Research on stress has progressed so rapidly in recent years that even our own Documentation Center has by now compiled an awe-inspiring 150,000 entries on stress and stress-related topics. The literature explosion has been even more considerable in connection with cancer research and psychosomatic medicine; this made it seem opportune in 1976 to present an overview of the entire field as it relates to virtually every facet of life in health and disease. [1] However, new developments in stress research continue to occur almost every day, and this creates a pressing need for annual overviews of the latest findings of our colleagues in this field. [2]

By way of an introduction, let us therefore deal with stress and the mind, at the same time stating our definitions of the basic concepts involved. Our first publication on stress and the general adaptation syndrome (G.A.S.) appeared in 1936 under the title "A syndrome produced by diverse nocuous agents." [3] Although it described our first primitive experiments on the stress concept more than 40 years ago and represented the very beginning of research in the field, it nonetheless holds true even today when we

Hans Selye • President, International Institute of Stress, University of Montreal, Montreal, Quebec H3C 3J7, Canada.

consider that the present definition of stress in biology contains much of the essence of those few original remarks on "the wear and tear of the body." Today, biologic stress is defined in most textbooks as "the nonspecific response of the body to any demand made upon it."

This rephrased definition was necessitated because, as time went by and more refined technology became available, it was noted that even happy circumstances, such as great pleasure, joy, or success, and healthy muscular exercise also trigger the same stereotyped stress response with the characteristic transmission of hypothalamic impulses to the pituitary for the mobilization of ACTH, corticoids, and other stress hormones, which is closely connected with Cannon's emergency "fight or flight" reaction accompanied by a massive autonomic discharge. Good stress, or *eustress* as we prefer to call it, is by definition agreeable, but if sudden and very intense, it can kill instantly, presumably as a result of cardiac fibrillation.

Each stressor or stress-producing agent, however, also elicits specific effects, depending upon its specific properties or characteristics, and these specific actions will in turn modify the nonspecific (stress) response of the organism. Furthermore, even the same stressor can exert different effects upon different people, because of their varying inherited and acquired stress susceptibility. The end result will depend, to a large extent, on the condition of the various organ systems, of which the weakest will naturally break down first. Thus, stress accompanies all disease phenomena and, in fact, all activities in life, but when the organism is exposed to any degree of stress incompatible with possibilities of adequate resistance or adaptation, stress can produce disease. In fact, stress is associated with every disease, although in some it plays a very small, and in others a very large role. And since stress is sometimes primarily responsible for the production of the most varied diseases, its predominant influence has led to such popular expressions as "stress diseases" or "diseases of adaptation," notably stress ulcers,[4] stress-induced disturbances of the cardiovascular system[5] or of the gastrointestinal tract,[4] neuropsychiatric disorders,[6] and allergies, to name a few. A certain predisposition is necessary in all of these maladies, and the same is true of cancer, in which the role of stress has been studied extensively but is still far from clear.

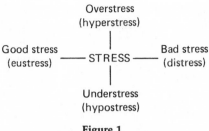

Figure 1

It could be said that biologic stress has four basic variations, although in their most characteristic nonspecific manifestations, they all depend upon the central phenomenon of stress itself.[7] This may be illustrated as shown in Figure 1.

The basic goal of a biologic code of behavior is therefore to strike a balance between the equally destructive forces of hypo- and hyperstress (in agreement with each individual's natural stress level) and to find as much eustress as possible, while minimizing distress. All these points have been described at length in earlier monographs.[1, 7-9]

Stress and cancer are related essentially in three ways: (1) cancer can produce considerable stress in patients; (2) stress can cause or aggravate cancer; and (3) stress can inhibit or even prevent cancer. However, before we go into a discussion of these points, we should say just a few words about the history of the relationship between psychologic factors influencing malignancy.

As early as 1759, Sir Richard Guy[10] suspected that cancer of the breast was particularly predominant among women showing hysteric and nervous signs of distress, especially melancholy. Two of his case reports described carcinoma of the breast in women following death of a child or imprisonment.

In 1885, the eminent American physician Willard Parker[11] noted that grief is especially frequent in the immediate history of patients with breast cancer. Two years later, Ephraim Cutter[12] observed that "mental depression is too often an element in cancerous cases to be overlooked." Amussat[13] in France and Paget[14] in England made similar observations at about the same time in the 19th century. Several researchers, whose work has been reviewed more recently,[15] expressed essentially similar ideas in the 18th and 19th centuries; and it appears that among their patients, the most frequently observed precursors were: "(1) loss of a significant figure (as a parent, child, spouse, etc.) through death or separation; (2) frustration of significant life situations and goals; and (3) a tendency toward despair, hopelessness, and grief when encountering stress, frustration, and/or loss."

Although none of them has been definitely proved, all these findings suggest that distress is a predisposing element in carcinogenesis; but it is somewhat artificial to discuss the predisposing actions of stress completely apart from its preventive or curative effects, because (depending upon conditions) it appears that stress can both promote and inhibit the formation of neoplasms.

It would seem opportune in the frame of this volume to outline the most extensively studied interrelations between stress, cancer, and the mind and to explore the most promising avenues for further research. On the basis of our own observations and literature studies, these appear to be the following:

(1) Malignant neoplasms undoubtedly elicit the typical manifestations of the G.A.S. (or stress syndrome) both in animals and in man.[16-20] For example, they produce hypertrophy and morphologic signs of hyperactivity in the adrenal cortex, an increase in plasma and urinary corticoids as well as their metabolites, involution of the thymicolymphatic apparatus, etc.[16-18, 20] They are also accompanied by the characteristic psychological responses to chronic stress.[19]

In leukemic strains of mice, fighting among males allegedly tends to delay the development of the disease, presumably through increased glucocorticoid production.[21] However, these claims have been contradicted by other investigators[22-26] and, in any event, not all types of neoplastic tissue react the same way. Indeed, according to certain authors,[27] stress enhances the development of metastases in experimental tumor-bearing animals.

There is also some evidence suggesting that, in mice, stressors capable of causing thymicolymphatic involution produce similar regressive changes in malignant tissue, although to a much lesser extent.[28]

(2) Exposure to a variety of stressors can induce malignant growths, especially in predisposed species under certain conditions.[29] This is true both of topically-applied and of systemic stressors. The evidence supporting the contention that local stress

can produce local tumorigenesis at the site of its application is particularly convincing.[1] The examples of chronic topical irritation—for example, of the lips by a pipe, the uterine cervix by pessaries, the skin by chronic irradiation with sunlight or heat—support this view on the basis of clinical observations. In addition, animal experiments have shown that chronic irritation with a variety of stimuli can elicit local neoplastic changes. In many of our own investigations, the introduction of irritants into a granuloma pouch in the rat caused subcutaneous sarcomas.[30] Similar observations were made even by the implantation of chemically-inert pyrex rings in the same species. Undoubtedly, here, we are dealing with nonspecific—that is, stressor—effects, not with those of specific carcinogens.[1]

(3) Considerably less evidence supports the assumption that systemic stress can influence tumorigenesis.[31] Undoubtedly, the glucocorticoids secreted upon exposure to stress do exert a moderate carcinolytic effect, and of course, the stress-induced changes in the immunologic system may also influence resistance to neoplasia.[32–36]

Stress caused by avoidance learning of high-frequency sound has no significant effect upon the development of malignant tumors induced in mice by polyoma virus.[37] On the other hand, in rats, restraint definitely increased susceptibility to the tumorigenic action of murine sarcoma virus.[34]

In rats, psychogenic stress allegedly inhibits the growth of most transplanted and chemically-induced tumors—a change that has been described as "characteristic of the stage of resistance of the G.A.S."[38]

Considerable literature has accumulated concerning the relationship between cancer and the mind. The interpretation of most of the reports is extremely difficult and subject to doubt. It has even been claimed that, under certain conditions, neoplasms can result from psychosomatic reactions in that certain predisposing personality characteristics and emotional states may play a significant role in the development, site, and course of cancer. On the other hand, regression of malignancies as a consequence of the patient's strong will to survive has also been postulated, but there is little tangible evidence to support such a view. Perhaps the most pressing task in this connection is to develop a code of behavior among patients with incurable malignancies and to train medical personnel in the techniques of making these trying times as tolerable as possible, both to the patients and to their relatives.

Perhaps a few recent references deserve special mention here. For example, in their latest volume, *Imagery of Cancer,* Achterberg and Lawlis[39] developed a model on the basis of our work on the stress of life[9] and formulated it in the following terms: "The emotions accompanying stress—fear, anxiety, and depression—are reflected in limbic system activity, which directly involves hypothalamic and pituitary function. The pituitary, the body's master gland, regulates all hormonal activity. Furthermore, imbalances in hormonal activity have frequently been demonstrated to be connected to increases in malignant growth. Oversecretion of the adrenal has been particularly noted to affect the thymus and lymph nodes and subsequently the white blood cells. Stress can thus be viewed as having a twofold influence on the malignant process: (1) the production of abnormal cells increases, and (2) the capability of the body to destroy these cells is diminished. Imagery moving in a positive direction may serve to alleviate the disruptive emotional condition and thereby intervene in the stress–disease–stress cycle."

This dual role of stress in inhibiting or promoting the development of cancer is shown, for example, by the observations of Charles Weinstock[40] on electroshock therapy. He concludes that "ECT and insulin coma appear quite regularly to bring approximately simultaneous marked beneficial effects on the patients' depression and cancer."

Eugene P. Pendergrass[41] summed up his opinion by stating "I personally have observed cancer patients who have undergone successful treatment and were living and well for years. Then an emotional stress such as the death of a son in World War II, the infidelity of a daughter-in-law, or the burden of long unemployment seem to have been precipitating factors in the reactivation of their disease which resulted in death. . . . There is solid evidence that the course of disease in general is affected by emotional distress."

Finally, we should mention a report of a novel and insufficiently studied aspect of severe sustained emotional stress and cancer, in which an enormous number of personal observations and large groups of statistically analyzed findings in various strata of the American population are discussed in relation to the effect of emotional stress upon cancer. [42] The conclusion is reached that, first of all, a person must be predisposed to carcinogenesis, but if this is the case, a severe distress can trigger the disease, whereas various educational measures can be extremely effective in inhibiting its progress. [42]

Other investigations worthy of reading in this connection are "Belief systems and management of the emotional aspects of malignancy," [43] "Suicide, cancer and depression," [44] "Grief as a disease process," [45] "Psychosomatic factors in the etiology of neoplasms," [46] "Psychological problems in terminal cancer management," [47] "Adjustment to cancer: A psychosocial and rehabilitative perspective," [48] and "Psychology of the exceptional cancer patient: A description of patients who outlive predicted life expectancies." [49]

In this brief review chapter, we wanted merely to outline the main correlations between stress, cancer, and the mind, and give access to the literature dealing with these subjects. It would be perfectly hopeless to discuss these complex and still unresolved matters from every point of view in a constructive manner, but it is hoped that the interested reader will find it useful to have access to data on virtually every aspect of cancer as a disease of adaptation, which in most cases is dependent upon some triggering factor.* This may be one of the well-known carcinogenic agents, such as X-irradiation, chemical carcinogens, smoking, etc., but perhaps most frequently stress plays a decisive role in it.

References

1. Selye, H. *Stress in Health and Disease*. Reading, Mass.: Butterworth, 1976.
2. Selye, H. *Selye's Guide to Stress Research*. New York: Van Nostrand Reinhold, in press.
3. Selye, H. A syndrome produced by diverse nocuous agents. *Nature (London)* 138:32, 1936.
4. Selye, H. Stress as a cause and consequence of peptic ulcers. Nutley, N.J.: *Roche Psychiatric Service Institute*, in press.

*A complete list of all pertinent papers to date may be obtained through the Documentation Service by writing to the Executive Director, International Institute of Stress, 2900 Boulevard Edouard-Montpetit, Montreal, Quebec H3C 3J7, Canada.

5. Selye, H. Stress and cardiovascular disease. *Cardiovas. Med.*, in press.
6. Selye, H. *Psychosocial implications of the stress concept.* In: T. Manschreck (Ed.), *The Massachusetts General Hospital Series on Psychiatric Medicine.* New York: Elsevier North-Holland, in press.
7. Selye, H. *The Stress of My Life.* Toronto: McClelland & Stewart, 1977. Revised updated edition, New York: Van Nostrand Reinhold, in press.
8. Selye, H. *Stress Without Distress.* New York: J. B. Lippincott, 1974.
9. Selye, H. *The Stress of Life.* 1st edition, New York: McGraw-Hill, 1956. 2nd edition, New York: McGraw-Hill, 1976.
10. Guy, R. *An Essay on Scirrhus Tumors and Cancers.* London: J. & A. Churchill, 1759.
11. Parker, W. *Cancer. A Study of 397 Cases of Cancer of the Female Breast.* New York: G. P. Putnam & Sons, 1885.
12. Cutter, E. Diet on cancer. *Albany Med. J.*8:218–251, July–August, 1887.
13. Amussat, J. Z. *Quelques Réflexions sur la Curabilité du Cancer.* Paris: E. Thunot, 1854.
14. Paget, J. *Surgical Pathology.* London: Longmans Green, 1870.
15. Kowal, S. J. Emotions as a cause of cancer. *Psychoanal. Rev.*42:217–227, 1955.
16. McEuen, C. S., and Selye, H. Histologic changes in the adrenals of tumor-bearing rats. *Am. J. Med. Sci.*189:423–424, 1935.
17. Hilf, R., Burnett, F. F., and Borman, A. The effect of Sarcoma 180 and other stressing agents upon adrenal and plasma corticosterone in mice. *Cancer Res.*20:1389–1393, 1960.
18. Hilf, R., Breuer, C., and Borman, A. The effect of Sarcoma 180 and other stressing agents upon adrenal adenine nucleotide-metabolizing enzymes. *Cancer Res.*21:1439–1444, 1961.
19. Moore, D. C., Holton, C. P., and Marten, G. W. Psychologic problems in the management of adolescents with malignancy. Experiences with 182 patients. *Clin. Pediatr.*8:464–473, 1969.
20. Ertl, N. "Systemic effects" during the growth of malignant experimental tumors. *Oncologia (Basel)*27:415–429, 1973.
21. Lemonde, P. Influence of fighting on leukemia in mice. *Proc. Soc. Exp. Biol. Med.*102:292–295, 1959.
22. Sławikowski, G. J. M. Tumor development in adrenalectomized rats given inoculations of aged tumor cells after surgical stress. *Cancer Res.*20:316–320, 1960.
23. Griffiths, J. D., and Hoppe, E. Effect of metabolic "stress" on development of tumor following inoculation of Walker carcinosarcoma cells. *Proc. Soc. Exp. Biol. Med.*104:467–469, 1960.
24. Gottfried, B., and Molomut, N. The influence of surgical trauma on the growth of tumor. An experimental evaluation. *J. Int. Coll. Surg.*36:Section 1, 596–602, 1961.
25. Gottfried, B., and Molomut, N. Effects of surgical trauma and other environmental stressors on tumor growth and wound healing. *Acta Unio. Int. Cancr.*20:1617–1620, 1964.
26. Pradhan, S. N., and Ray, P. Effects of stress on growth of transplanted and 7,12-dimethylbenz[α]anthracene-induced tumors and their modification by psychotropic drugs. *J. Natl. Cancer Inst.*53:1241–1245, 1974.
27. Cole, W. H. The mechanisms of spread of cancer. *Surg. Gynec. Obstet.*137:853–871, 1973.

28. Bass, A. D., and Feigelson, M. Response of normal and malignant lymphoid tissue to non-specific tissue damage. *Proc. Soc. Exp. Biol. Med*69:339–341, 1948.
29. Stern, J. A., Winokur, G., Graham, D. T, and Lefton, R. Effect of enforced activity stress on the development of experimental papillomas in mice. *J. Natl. Cancer Inst.*23:1013–1018, 1959.
30. Selye, H. An experimental model illustrating the pathogenesis of the diseases of adaptation. *J. Clin. Endocrinol. Metab.*14:997–1005, 1954.
31. Arasa, F. La problemática del cáncer vista por un médico humanista. *Folia Clin. Int. (Barcelona)*24:547–557, 1974.
32. Solomon, G. F. Emotions, stress, the central nervous system, and immunity. *Ann. N.Y. Acad. Sci.*164:335–343, 1969.
33. Amkraut, A. A., Solomon, G. F., Kasper, P., and Purdue, A. Stress and hormonal intervention in the graft-versus-host response. *Adv. Exp. Med. Biol.*29:667–674, 1973.
34. Seifter, E., Rettura, G., Zisblatt, M., Levenson, S. M., Levine, N., Davidson, A., and Seifter, J. Enhancement of tumor development in physically-stressed mice inoculated with an oncogenic virus. *Experientia*29:1379–1382, 1973.
35. Spackman, D., and Riley, V. Increased corticosterone, a factor in LDH-virus induced alterations of immunological responses in mice. *Proc. Amer. Assoc. Cancer Res.*15:143, 1974.
36. Howard, R. J., and Simmons, R. L. Acquired immunologic deficiencies after trauma and surgical procedures. *Surg. Gynec. Obstet.*139:771–782, 1974.
37. Rasmussen, A. F., Hildemann, W. H., and Sellers, M. Malignancy of polyoma virus infection in mice in relation to stress. *J. Natl. Cancer Inst*30:101–112, 1963.
38. Ray, P., and Pradhan, S. N. Brief communication: Growth of transplanted and induced tumors in rats under a schedule of punished behavior. *J. Natl. Cancer Inst.*52:575–577, 1974.
39. Achterberg, J., and Lawlis, G. F. *Imagery of Cancer*. Champaign, Ill.: Institute for Personality & Ability Testing, 1978.
40. Weinstock, C. Recent progress in cancer psychobiology and psychiatry. *J. Amer. Soc. Psychosom. Dent. Med*24:4–14, 1977.
41. Pendergrass, E. Presidential address to American Cancer Society Meeting, 1959.
42. Reichel, S. *Severe Sustained Emotional Stress and Cancer*. S. M. Reichel, 1977.
43. Simonton, O. C., and Simonton, S. S. Belief systems and management of the emotional aspects of malignancy. *J. Trans. Psychol*7:29–47, 1975.
44. Whitlock, F. A. Suicide, cancer and depression. *Brit. J. Psychiat*132:269–274, 1978.
45. Fredrick, J. F. Grief as a disease process. *Omega (Westport, Conn.)*7:297–305, 1977.
46. Watson, C. G., and Schuld, D. Psychosomatic factors in the etiology of neoplasms. *J. Cons. Clin. Psychol*45:455–461, 1977.
47. Rothenberg, A. Psychological problems in terminal cancer management. *Cancer (Philadelphia)*14:1063–1073, 1961.
48. McCollum, P. S. Adjustment to cancer: A psychosocial and rehabilitative perspective. *Rehabil. Council Bull.*21:216–223, 1978.
49. Achterberg, Matthews, S., and Simonton, O. C. Psychology of the exceptional cancer patient: A description of patients who outlive predicted life expectancies. *Psychother. Theory Res. Pract.* June 21:1–21, 1976.

2

The Possible Effects of Emotional Stress on Cancer Mediated through the Immune System

Martin G. Lewis, M.D., M.R.C. [Path.], and Terence M. Phillips, Ph.D., A.R.I.C.

Introduction

The complex pathological changes which we collectively call cancer present a series of complicated interactions within the interrelated systems of the body. It is not unreasonable, therefore, that consideration should be given to the possible ways in which the malignant process and the higher centers of the nervous system interact. Although a good deal of attention has been given to the consequences of malignancy on the central nervous system apart from the mechanical effects of metastasis, there is a growing awareness that the areas of the brain collectively concerned with emotions may in turn modify the development and progression of cancer. It is this latter aspect which will be considered in this paper.

Martin G. Lewis • Chairman, Department of Pathology, Georgetown University School of Medicine and Dentistry, Washington, D.C. 20007. Terence M. Phillips • Georgetown University School of Medicine and Dentistry, Washington, D.C. 20007.

There are numerous potential ways in which a malignant tumor can be modified. These include alterations in the blood supply, general nutrition, the genetic makeup of the individual, the inherent growth pattern of the tumor itself, and particularly the endocrine system. The possibility, however, that immunological changes may also be involved in the malignant process has led to a considerable interest in this aspect of host–tumor relationships. It has been the experience of those dealing with cancer both in humans and in experimental animals for a number of years that cancer is not a uniform phenomenon.[1] It is an everyday experience that patients with identical cancers at identical sites do not react identically. It is also often noted that some form of emotional disturbance may precede the appearance of clinical cancer in humans; and although these phenomena have been difficult to document and characterize, sufficient evidence has accumulated clearly showing this to be a relationship not to be lightly dismissed. Malignant tumors do not behave as simple tissue cultures. A series of dynamic interactions between the tumor and various forms of host resistance can occur. It is the purpose of this paper to consider whether emotional stress can influence the behavior of malignant tumors and whether this effect is mediated through some form of immune interaction between the tumor and the higher centers of the brain.

The Immune System and Cancer

The suggestion that immunological reactions may occur in cancer patients or modify the progression of tumors is by no means a new one. In 1900, Paul Ehrlich giving the Croonian Lecture to the Royal Society in London made the statement: "The idea has already been mooted by von Dungen of attacking epithelium new formations, particularly carcinoma, by means of specific anti-epithelial serum."[2] In the ensuing years, both experimenters with animals and those studying humans gathered a considerable body of data suggesting that some forms of immune reaction occur in patients with malignancy and tumor-bearing animals. This situation has reached a point within the past few years in which it is now possible to measure both antibody and cell-mediated immune reactions in human and animals directed against their growing tumors.[3] It has also been possible in many animal models to modify the growth of tumors by altering the immune response. This can result in both enhancement or rejection of the tumors by suitable immune manipulations.[4] In the human, the evidence is more circumstantial but still fairly convincing, and immunotherapy of cancer has now become at least one of the various adjuncts to the treatment of this disease.[5] It is clear, however, that an explanation is still needed as to why an immune system that apparently recognizes a tumor as foreign should not in every case successfully reject that tumor or at least prevent its growth. There have been a number of theories put forward to answer this question. The most attractive of these are concerned with some form of internal blockade or abnormal regulation of the immune response allowing the tumor to grow in the face of a confused host resistance.[6,7] It is clear that various largely unexplored factors—including endocrine abnormalities and emotional stress—may play a vital role in this problem of immune regulation and derangement.

Stress and the Immune System

Although it has for many years been the experience of medical practitioners that severe emotional disturbance can lead to illness, the exact mechanism to explain this interaction has been explored seriously only in recent years.[8-10] There have been numerous observations that many human pathological conditions are preceded by severe emotional disturbance of one type or another. These conditions include those clearly related to the immune system—particularly autoimmunity, a situation where the immune system in a sense attacks its own host.[11] As a result of these observations, new experimental approaches have been proposed for dealing with this problem. There is a growing awareness that manipulations of certain centers of the brain—either directly or via emotional stress—can modify measurable aspects of the immune response, and that this can be detected in antibody production and in terms of cell-mediated immunity.[12] This opens up numerous opportunities for further exploration, and also presents the possibility of relating this abnormal immune response to disease, including malignancy.

Stress, Immunity, and Cancer

As a result of the foregoing developments, it is not surprising that there have been several reports indicating a direct link between emotional stress and cancer mediated through the immune system. This has been shown indirectly by *in vitro* studies of humans where abnormal immune responses have been measured in patients suffering emotional disturbances.[12] Perhaps more convincingly, it has been possible to produce in experimental animals emotional stress conditions which can then be shown to modify the growth and spread of transplantable or chemically induced tumors.[13–16] This has further been shown to be related to abnormal immune responses as measured by *in vivo* and *in vitro* test systems in the experimental animals.[17] For instance, the placing of a cat in the presence of a cage of mice resulted in an alteration in the immune responses to infections with certain parasites.[18] More direct approaches have been shown in experiments where the hypothalamus has been stimulated electronically and direct alterations in antibody and cell-mediated immune responses were noted.[19]

Recent developments in the field of abnormal immune reactions in cancer patients and experimental animals have led to the concept of an abnormal immune regulation with immune derangement. This concept holds that chronic antigenic stimulation produced by the persistence of the growing tumor gives rise to a series of changes, including the presence of immune complexes, anti-antibodies, and subsequent production of cell-mediated anergy.[20] These same manifestations of immune derangement are seen in autoimmune diseases, chronic bacterial infections, and parasitic infestations, bringing malignancy into line with these disorders. Some years ago, Jerne suggested that one of the ways of explaining the regulation of the immune response was to regard the system as a network in which positive and negative feedback control occurred. [21] Therefore, if one argues that the immune system is designed to respond to antigenic stimulation—but on the basis of its being a short-lived experience—then the persistence of the antigenic stimulation would be expected to lead to a breakdown of this self-regulatory control. In this sense, the immune system is controlled in a manner similar to that of the endocrine and coagulation systems. We have already suggested that changes in emotional status or physical stimulation of areas of the hypothalamus and related areas can result in alterations of immune response. It is also known that the same areas control to some extent the regulation of the endocrine system. It would not be unreasonable to suggest that emotional changes might well produce an effect on the malignant process through this abnormal regulation of immune responses.

Summary and Conclusion

It is clear, therefore, that from historical and circumstantial evidence—and in more recent times through experimental data and *in vitro* assays—that a direct link between abnormal immune responses, the growth of malignant tumors, and various forms of emotional disturbance and stress exists. Although this field and its links are certainly in an early phase of development, methods now exist both in laboratories and clinics which we hope will permit more detailed and more accurate assessment of this complicated interaction. That a self-regulatory system is involved makes the problem considerably more difficult than first imagined. Now, the clear prospect that an even more complex regulatory system— namely, the brain—is also involved adds a further dimension to this problem. While this new dimension adds to the complexity of the problem, it also generates a great deal of excitement in an area of research heretofore well beyond the narrow limitations of the experimental laboratory. And yet, as Metchnikoff stated in 1905: "Science is very far from having said its last word, but advances already made are amply sufficient to dispel pessimism in so far as this has been suggested by the fear of the disease, the feeling that we are powerless in the struggle against it." [22]

References

1. Foulds, L. *Neoplastic Development*, Vol. 2. New York: Academic Press, 1975, p. 228.
2. Ehrlich, P. Croonian lecture on immunity with special reference to cell life. *Proc. Royal Soc. Med.*66:424, 1900.
3. Lewis, M. G. Immunology and the melanomas. *Curr. Top. Microbiol. Immunol.*63:49, 1974.
4. Vaage, J. Protective serum effects in tumor immunity. *Israel J. Med. Sci.*12:334, 1976.
5. Morton, D. L. Cancer immunotherapy: An overview. *Semin. Oncol.*1:297, 1974.
6. Jerry, L. M., Lewis, M. G., and Cano, P. O. Anergy, anti-antibodies and immune complex disease: A syndrome of disordered immune regulation in human cancer. In Martin, M., and Dionne, L. (Eds.), *Immunocancerology in Solid Tumors.* Québec: Septième Symposium de Cancérologie, Faculté de Médecine de l'Université Laval, 1976.
7. Lewis, M. G., Phillips, T. M., Rowden, G., and Jerry, L. M. Humoral immune reactions in cancer patients. In *Handbook of Cancer Immunology.* New York: Garland, 1977, p. 159.
8. Rahe, R. H. Subjects' recent life changes and their near-future illness susceptibility. *Adv. Psychosom. Med.*8:2,1972.
9. Jacobs, M. A., Spilken, A., and Norman, M. Relationship of life change, maladaptive aggression, and upper respiratory infection in male college students. *Psychosom. Med.*31:31, 1969.
10. Palmblad, P., Cantell, K., Strander, H., Froberg, J., Karlsson, C. G., Levi, L., Granstrom, M., and Unger, P. Stressor exposure and immunological response in man: Interferon-producing capacity and phagocytosis. *J. Psychol. Res.*20:193, 1976.
11. Soloman, G. F., Amkraut, A. A., and Kasper, P. Immunity, emotions and stress. *Ann. Clin. Res.*6:313, 1974.
12. Stein, M., Schiavi, R. C., and Camerino, M. Influence of brain and behavior on the immune system. *Science*191:435, 1976.
13. Van den Brenk, H. A. S., Stone, M. G., Kelly, H., and Sharpington, C. Lowering of innate resistance of the lungs to the growth of blood-borne cancer cells in states of topical and systemic stress. *Brit. J. Cancer*33:60, 1976.
14. Joãsoo, A., and McKenzie, J. M. Stress and the immune response in rats. *Int. Archs. Allergy Appl. Immunol.*50:659, 1976.
15. Peters, L. J., and Kelly, H. The influence of stress and stress hormones on the transplantability of a non-immunogenic syngeneic murine tumor. *Cancer*39:1482, 1977.
16. Ebbesen, P., and Rask-Kielsen, R. Influence of sex-segregated grouping and of inoculation of subcellular leukemic material on development of non-leukemic lesions in DBA/2, BALB/c, and CBA mice. *J. Nat. Cancer Inst.*39:917, 1967.
17. Monjan, A. A., and Collector, M. I. Stress-induced modulation of the immune response. *Science*196:307, 1977.
18. Hamilton, D. R. Immunosuppressive effects of predator induced stress in mice with acquired immunity to *Hymenolepis nana. J. Psychol. Res.*18:143, 1974.

19. Soloman, G. F., Amkraut, A. A., and Kasper, P. Immunity, emotions, and stress. With special reference to the mechanisms of stress effects on the immune system. *Psychother. Psychosom.*23:209, 1974.
20. Lewis, M. G., Hartmann, D., and Jerry, L. M. Antibodies and anti-antibodies in human malignancy: An expression of deranged immune regulation. *Ann. N.Y. Acad. Sci.*276:316, 1976.
21. Jerne, N. K. Immune regulation in a lymphocyte network. In Edelman, G. M. (Ed.), *Cellular Selection and Regulation in the Immune Response.* New York: Raven Press, p. 39, 1974.
22. Metchnikiff, E. Immunity in infective disease. Translated by F. G. Binnie. In *The Sources of Science Handbooks*, No. 61. New York and London: Johnson Reprint Corporation, p. 569, 1968.

3

Stress, Hormone Responses, and Cancer

G. M. Brown, M.D., Ph.D., J. Seggie, Ph.D., and P. Ettigi, M.D.

A wide variety of hormones are highly responsive to stressful stimulation. As we all know, the hallmark of stress is adrenal activation as first demonstrated by Selye for the adrenal cortex and by Cannon for the adrenal medulla (Mason, 1968). It is now known that release of corticosteroids from the adrenal gland is triggered by ACTH release from the anterior pituitary, which is in turn provoked by the release of corticotropin-releasing factor from the hypothalamus (James and Landon, 1968; Oken, 1967; Mason, 1968). The development of sensitive assay systems has led to the ability to measure all the anterior pituitary hormones in blood in man. It has now been shown that the patterns of release of many of these hormones are altered by stressful stimulation. In another series of

G. M. Brown • Chairman, Department of Neurosciences, McMaster University, Hamilton, Ontario L8S 4J9, Canada. J. Seggie • Department of Neurosciences, McMaster University, Hamilton, Ontario L8S 4J9, Canada. P. Ettigi • Department of Psychiatry, Medical College of Virginia, Richmond, Virginia 23298. Work described in this chapter was supported in part by Grant MT 4749 from the Medical Research Council of Canada and by Grant 729 from the Ontario Mental Health Foundation.

exciting developments, the hypothalamic factors controlling several of the anterior pituitary hormones have been isolated, characterized, and synthesized (Martin *et al.*, 1977).

Multiple Stress Hormone Responses

In addition to adrenocorticotropic hormone (ACTH), two other anterior pituitary hormones are highly stress-responsive: namely, growth hormone and prolactin (Brown, Seggie, and Feldman, 1977; Seggie and Brown, 1975; Seggie and Brown, 1976*b*; Brown and Reichlin, 1972; Sachar, 1975). In addition, it is known that thyrotropin (TSH) is increased in response to stressful stimuli and (LH) is released in response to surgical stress in male patients (Aono *et al.*, 1976; Guansing *et al.*, 1975). Moreover, a variety of studies too numerous to mention here indicate that there is pronounced adrenal medullary activation in response to stressful stimuli as well as activation of the posterior lobe of the pituitary (Martin *et al.*, 1977). It may thus be concluded that in response to acute stressful stimulation, there are multiple changes in hormone release (Figure 1).

Species Differences

It should be pointed out that there are certain important species differences in these responses. Thus in man and in monkey, growth hormone responds to stressful stimulation with

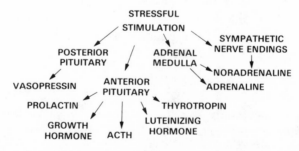

Figure 1. In response to stressful stimulation, there are multiple effects on hormone release involving sympathetic nerve endings, adrenal medulla, and both anterior and posterior lobes of the pituitary gland. ACTH: adrenocorticotropic hormone.

an acute increase which parallels the change in adrenal steroids seen in these species (Brown and Reichlin, 1972; Brown, Seggie, and Feldman, 1977). In contrast to the primate, rats show an acute lowering of blood growth hormone after stimulation (Brown and Martin, 1973; Seggie and Brown, 1975; Seggie and Brown, 1976a). This finding may be the most striking example of species differences but is far from the only such instance. One conclusion to be derived from these observations is that human studies are required in order to properly evaluate stress hormone responses in man. On the other hand, animal experimentation is essential for the elucidation of the neural and psychologic correlates of the response, and the overall pattern may well be similar in animals and man (Brown and Reichlin, 1972; Seggie and Brown, 1976a).

Factors Modulating Stress Responses

A number of factors other than stress alter the levels of pituitary hormones in the circulation. These factors are also known to interact with and modify the stress-responding mechanisms. Thus, the stress responses are superimposed upon resting levels which are anything but constant, and these stress responses are modified by many of the same factors which alter resting levels.

It has been known for some time that most hormone levels exhibit diurnal changes that are rhythmical in nature (Retiene, 1970). Adrenal steroid output exhibits a diurnal rhythm in the resting state in both man (Weitzman *et al.*, 1971) and rat (Critchlow *et al.*, 1963), thus providing a fluctuating baseline. Prolactin levels also have been reported to evince various 24-hour variations (Dunn *et al.*, 1972; Nokin *et al.*, 1972). However, in view of the very low and possibly diurnally variable threshold of sensitivity of prolactin levels to environmental stimulation, it has been questioned whether some of the variation seen in prolactin levels may be due to methodological artifacts (Seggie and Brown, 1976b). Growth hormone, too, has shown a diurnal rhythm in resting levels (Seggie and Brown, 1976a). It is now clearly known that the pattern of hormone response obtained following a given stimulus is dependent upon the point in the diurnal cycle at which the test challenge is imposed (Seggie and Brown, 1975; Brown and Martin, 1974).

Superimposed on the rhythmic 24-hour pattern of hormone release is a daily pattern of episodic bursts. For instance, human ACTH and cortisol secretion shows a diurnal variation that is composed of seven to nine episodic bursts during the 24-hour day (Weitzman et al., 1971). Growth hormone also is released in an episodic fashion with up to eight individual surges occurring in a 24-hour period. In addition, surge peaks are higher during the first part of sleep, thus contributing to an overall diurnal variation in growth hormone levels. Age also affects growth hormone surges with an increased number of surges occurring during puberty (Martin et al., 1977). A pattern of episodic secretion has also been observed for prolactin (Sassin et al., 1972), thyroid-stimulating hormone (Vanhaelst et al., 1972), and the gonadotropins (Boyar et al., 1972). Indeed, a pattern of episodic secretion has been found in all anterior pituitary hormones studied to date. The net result of this type of secretion is that the active secretion period for any one hormone may be quite brief and the standard error of average values will thus be very high.

In order for maximum information to be obtained from neuroendocrine measures, conditions of sampling must be controlled for time of day, as well as for a variety of other factors known to alter the levels such as the type of environmental and psychological stimulation conditions surrounding the sampling, sex, menstrual phase, age, stage of development of puberty, metabolic factors such as state of nutrition, pharmacological treatment, and perhaps even the season of the year. Adequate control of these factors has rarely been achieved, probably because of the lack of knowledge of these factors.

Neural Control

It was noted above that hormone secretion from the pituitary is in turn controlled by the release of hypothalamic factors from the hypothalamus. Since the speed of neural events is very rapid (being measured in milliseconds) while the speed of hormone responses is considerably slower (usually measured in minutes), it is obvious that stress-responding circuits could be localized at a distance from the hypothalamus and that they are not necessarily located within the hypothalamus. Investigations on neural regulation of hormone release in response to stress in experimental animals suggest that the ability to cope with stress may be dependent on a specific extrahypothalamic neural network.

Damage to the septal area of the limbic system in rats causes a behavior disturbance characterized by overreactivity to stimulation and a potentiation of the normal stress response pattern of both corticosterone and growth hormone without altering the characteristic diurnal rhythm and resting levels of either of these hormones (Seggie and Brown, 1976a). Thus, it appears that there is a central neural mechanism controlling responses to stress that is independent of those mechanisms responsible for the homeostatic control of hormone levels. Normal resting hormone responses are not necessarily disturbed even when there is extensive damage to this neural center. Preliminary data from ongoing work in another area of the limbic system lead to a similar set of conclusions. Rats subjected to destruction of various parts of the amygdala showed a concordance of their behavioral and hormonal responses to stressful stimuli similar to those animals with septal lesions. Animals were studied under similar conditions to those previously described for studies on the septal region (Seggie and Brown, 1976a). The data available up to now on the amygdala region of animals are shown in Table 1, with the previously published data on septal animals at the bottom of the Table. If the amygdala (or septal) lesion produces an animal that does not cope with the stimulus behaviorally, then an alteration in the hormone response is also found. In contrast, even in the face of massive damage to the amygdala or septum, no change in hormone levels is found under conditions of rest. Furthermore, when no behavior disturbance is found, there is no hormone abnormality. These findings suggest several hypotheses; for example, (1) the septum and the basolateral amygdala are an integral part of a neural network required for coping with stressful stimuli, i.e., nonhomeostatic needs are controlled by a specific neural network; (2) the corticomedial amygdala, although not required for coping with the stimuli used in these studies, may be required for coping with other environmental stimuli, i.e., the neural network for coping with stressful stimulation may be stimulus-specific. It is hoped that future work will

TABLE 1. Effects of Brain Lesions on Various
Hormone and Behavior Parameters

Area of brain damage	Behavior under stress	Resting 24-hour hormone levels	Hormone response to stress
Whole amygdala complex	—	Corticosterone, growth hormone, and prolacting all normal	—
Basolateral amygdala	Hyperreactive	Corticosterone, growth hormone, prolactin, and testosterone all normal	Corticosterone potentiated
Corticomedial amygdala	Normal	Corticosterone and prolactin normal	Corticosterone normal
Septum	Hyperreactive	Corticosterone, growth hormone, and prolactin all normal	Corticosterone and growth hormone potentiated

clarify this issue. For the present, one can only state that peripherally obtained hormone measures can be used as an index of centrally occurring events. Examining hormone responses in lesioned animals is a strategy which should permit mapping of the neural network involved in coping.

Hormone Alterations in Depression

Several studies have shown that psychological factors produce changes in a variety of endocrine parameters (Brown *et al.*, 1974; Sachar, 1975). Several psychiatric conditions such as affective disorders, anorexia nervosa, and premenstrual syndrome have been shown to have specific endocrine disturbances. For example, Ettigi and Brown (1977), reviewing neuroendocrine function in affective disorder, have documented alteration in the regulation of cortisol, growth hormone (GH), prolactin, thyroid-stimulating hormone (TSH), and luteinizing hormone (LH) in such patients (Table 2). Cortisol hypersecretion in depressed patients has been shown by monitoring plasma levels around the clock. This hypersecretion is characterized by increase in both number and magnitude of secretory episodes as well as a pervasive increase in plasma cortisol concentration which is elevated not only during the night as in normal subjects but also during the daytime when control subjects have very low levels. These increased bursts of cortisol secretion are related to increased episodic release of ACTH from the pituitary. GH response to insulin hypoglycemia has been shown to be lower in certain depressed patients compared to control subjects. GH response to thyrotropin-releasing hormone (TRH) is elevated in depressed patients when compared to controls. Depressed patients have also been reported to show an inadequate or lowered TSH response to TRH in comparison to healthy control subjects. One group of workers has shown diminished plasma LH levels in depressed postmenopausal women. Evidence in relation to prolactin is uncertain as one group has shown the prolactin response to TRH to be elevated while another has reported a diminished response in depressed patients.

Comparison of the hormonal changes occurring following acute stressful stimulation with those occurring with endogenous depression establishes that the alterations differ and are specific to the condition.

Cancer and Stress

Several workers have investigated the relation of various psychological mechanisms such as defenses, conflicts, life stresses,

TABLE 2. Hormonal Changes Following Acute Stress as Compared to Endogenous Depression

Hormone	Acute stress	Endogenous depression
ACTH	Increase	Increased output, flattened diurnal variation
		Reduced response to dexamethasone
GH	Increase	Reduced response to hypoglycemia
		Responds after TRH
Prolactin	Increase	Results conflict
TSH	Increase	Decreased response to TRH

and life styles as contributing factors in the etiology of cancer (see reviews by Leshan and Worthington, 1956; Crisp, 1970; Abse *et al.*, 1974; Brown *et al.*, 1974). The idea that cancer may occur in certain personality types has been current since the days of Galen, who observed cancer to be more frequent in "melancholic" rather than "sanguine" women (Kowal, 1955). Over the years, several anecdotal observations have been made about the psychosomatic aspects of malignancy. Kissen *et al.* (1969) have shown by careful, experimentally-controlled studies that people with (lung) cancer showed poor and restricted outlets for emotional discharge even before the onset of cancer. Bahnson *et al.* (1969) and Bahnson (1976), studying the ego defense mechanisms of cancer patients, found that their data support the presence of extreme repression and denial in such patients. Using a variety of techniques such as detailed developmental and case history taking, projective tests, and personality inventories, several groups of workers have studied the relation between personality factors and cancer. On examining this body of work, the various reviews do point out with some degree of consistency that certain personality factors tend to be characteristic of cancer patients even prior to onset of illness. Some of these personality factors are denial and repression; impaired self-awareness and introspective capacity; poor outlet for emotional discharge; little expression of aggression; self-sacrificing and self-blaming tendency; and predisposition for experiencing hopelessness and despair (Abse *et al.*, 1974). Important precipitating psychological factors that have been listed are (1) the patient's loss of an important relationship prior to the development of the tumor; (2) the cancer patient's inability to express hostile feelings and emotions; (3) presence of unresolved tension concerning parental figure (Leshan and Worthington, 1956). In spite of several studies suggesting the presence of characteristic defenses and emotionality in patients with cancer, there has been little evidence suggesting that there is a difference in life style which would serve to distinguish cancer-prone personalities from other personalities (Abse *et al.*, 1974). It has been pointed out—and one still has to bear in mind—that these physical and psychological manifestations in cancer patients may be coincidental, i.e., stemming from different causes. It is also possible that a single underlying neural or endocrine factor may cause both emotional disturbance and cancer, and that stress may be a causative factor in the development of cancer through the intermediary of the stress hormones (Meerloo, 1954). Psychological disturbance may so disturb the body chemistry that cancer *in situ* may become a malignant tumor.

One route through which stress hormones may influence cancer is via the immune system. It has been known for years that stress can influence immunity. One example of this is a recent study which shows that immunity can be conditioned (Ader and Cohen, 1975). Recently, it has been shown that growth hormone receptors exist on lymphocytes (Lesniak *et al.*, 1974). Lymphocytes in turn are an integral part of the immune defenses which are thought to be involved in cancer. Since there is a mechanism by which the brain can influence immunity and since at least one stress hormone may influence the immune system, it is possible that stress influences immunity via a hormonal route. If this is so, it is possible that stress hormones acting via the immune system can influence either the appearance or the cause of cancer. It is therefore of some interest that in recent years reports on the effect of hormones on cancer have been increasing in number (Stern *et al.*, 1969). For example, prolactin has been found to have an effect on the progress of certain types of breast cancer (Ettigi *et al.*, 1973) while estrogens in the form of replacement therapy have been incriminated as a cause of endometrial cancer (Mack *et al.*, 1976). In these instances, effects are due to action of the hormones at target tissues, rather than by acting on immune systems. There may well be other instances in which hormones produce effects by an action on immune processes.

Conclusion

In order to know the relationship of ACTH, growth hormone, prolactin, and other stress hormones to cancer, it will be necessary to study them in some detail. A computer search of the literature which we conducted in the fall of 1977 revealed few significant studies in this area. The field appears largely to be virgin territory which we recommend to those who are interested in cancer.

References

Abse, D. W., Wilkins, M. M., van de Castle, R. L., Buston, W. D., Demans, J. P.,
    Brown, R. S., and Kirschner, L. G. Personality and behavioural characteristics of
    lung cancer patients. *J. Psychosom. Res.*18:101–113, 1974.
Ader, R., and Cohen, N. Behaviourally conditioned immunosuppression. *Psycho-
    som. Med.*37:333–348, 1975.
Aono, T., Kurachi, K., Miyata, M., Nakasima, A., Koshiyama, K., Uojumi, T., and
    Matsumoto, K. Influence of surgical stress under general anaesthesia on serum
    gonadotropin levels in male and female patients. *J. Clin. Endocrinol.
    Metab.*42:144–148, 1976.
Bahnson, C. B. Emotional and personality characteristics of cancer patients. In: A.
    E. Sutnick and P. F. Engstrom (Eds.), *Oncologic Medicine, Clinical Topics and
    Practical Management.* Baltimore: University Park Press, 1976, pp. 357–378.
Bahnson, M. B., and Bahnson, C. B. Ego defenses in cancer patients. *Ann. N.Y.
    Acad. Sci.*164:546, 1969.
Boyar, R., Perilow, M., Hellman, L., Kopen, S., Weitzman, E. Twenty-four hour
    pattern of luteinizing hormone secretion in normal men with sleep stage record-
    ing. *J. Clin. Endocrinol. Metab.*35:73–81, 1972.
Brown, G. M., and Reichlin, S. Psychologic and neural regulation of GH secretion.
    *Psychosom. Med.*34:45–61, 1972.
Brown, G. M., and Martin, J. B. Corticosterone, prolactin and growth hormone.
    Responses to handling and new environment in the rat. *Psychosom. Med.*36:241–
    247, 1974.
Brown, J. H., Varsamisj, J., Toews, J., and Shane, M. Psychiatry and oncology: A
    review. *Can. Psychiatr. Assoc. J.*19:219, 1974.
Brown, G. M., Seggie, J., and Feldman, J. Effect of psychosocial stimuli and limbic
    lesions on prolactin at rest and following stress. *Clin. Endocrinol. (Oxford)* 6
    (suppl.):29s–41s, 1977.
Crisp, A. H. Some psychosomatic aspects of neoplasia. *Br. J. Med. Psychol.*43:313–
    331, 1970.
Critchlow, V., Liebelt, R. A., Bar-Sela, M., Mountcastle, W., and Lipscomb, H. C.
    Sex differences in resting pituitary-adrenal function in the rat. *Am. J.
    Psychol.*205:807–815, 1963.
Dunn, J., Arimura, A., and Scheving, L. Effect of stress on Circadian periodicity in
    serum LH and prolactin. *Endocrinology*90:29–33, 1972.
Ettigi, P., Lal, S., and Friesen, H. G. Prolactin, phenothiazines, admission to mental
    hospital and carcinoma of the breast. *Lancet*2:266–267, 1973.
Ettigi, P. G., and Brown, G. M. Psychoneuroendocrinology of affective disorder:
    An overview. *Am. J. Psychiatry*134:493–501, 1977.
Guansing, A.R., Leung, Y., Ajlouni, K., and Kagen, T. C. The Effect of hypo-
    glycemia on TSH release in man. *J. Clin. Endocrinol. Metab.*40:755–758, 1975.
James, V. H. T., and Landon, J. *The Investigation of Hypothalamic-Pituitary-Adrenal
    Function.* Cambridge: University Press, 311, 1968.
Katz, J., Gallagher, T., Hellman, L., Sachar, E., and Weiner, H. Psychoendocrine
    considerations in cancer of the breast. *Ann. N.Y. Acad. Sci.*164:509–515, 1969.
Kissen, D. M., Brown, R. I. F., and Kissen, M. A. A further report on personality
    and psychosocial factors in lung cancer. *Ann. N.Y. Acad. Sci.*164:535, 1969.
Kowal, S. J. Emotions as a cause of cancer: 18th and 19th century contributions.
    *Psychoanal. Rev.*42:217, 1955.

Leshan, L. L., and Worthington, R. E. Personality as a factor in the pathogenesis of cancer: A review of literature. *Br. J. Med. Psychol.* 29:49–56, 1956.

Lesniak, M. A., Gorden, P., Roth, J., and Gavin, J. R. Binding of ^{125}I-human growth hormone to specific receptors in human cultured lymphocytes. *J. Biol. Chem* 249:1661–1667, 1974.

Mack, T. M., Pike, M. C. Henderson, B., Pfeffer, R., Gerkins, V., Arthur, M., and Brown, S. Estrogens and endometrial cancer in a retirement community. *New Eng. J. Med.* 294:1262–1267, 1976.

Martin, J. B. Brain regulation of growth hormone secretion. In: Martini L., and Ganong, W. F. (Eds.), *Frontiers in Neuroendocrinology, Vol. 4.* New York: Raven Press, 1976.

Martin, J. B., Reichlin, S., and Brown, G. M. *Clinical Neuroendocrinology, Vol. 14.* Contemporary Neurology Series. Philadelphia: F. A. Davis, 410, 1977.

Mason, J. A review of psychoendocrine research on the pituitary-adrenal-cortical system. *Psychosom. Med.* 30:576–607, 1968.

Meerloo, J. A. M. Psychological implication of malignant growth. *Br. J. Med. Psychol.* 27:210–215, 1954.

Nokin, J., Vekemans, M., L'Hermite, M., and Robyn, C. Circadian periodicity of serum prolactin concentration in man. *Br. Med. J.* 3:561–562, 1972.

Oken, D. The psychophysiology and psychoendocrinology of stress and emotion. In: M. Appley, and R. Turnbull (Eds.), *Psychological Stress.* New York: Appleton-Century-Crofts, 1967.

Retiene, K. Control of circadian periodicities in pituitary function. In: L. Martini, M. Motta, and F. Fraschinie (Eds.), *The Hypothalamus.* New York: Academic Press, 1970.

Sachar, E. J. Hormonal changes in stress and mental illness. *Hosp. Pract.* 10:49–55, 1975.

Sassin, J. F., Frantz, A. G., Weitzman, E. D., and Kapen, S. Human prolactin: 24 hour pattern with increased release during sleep. *Science* 177:1205–1207, 1972.

Seggie, J., and Brown, G. M. Stress response patterns of plasma corticosterone, prolactin and growth hormone in the rat following handling or exposure to novel environment. *Can. J. Physiol. Pharmacol.* 53:629–637, 1975.

Seggie, J., and Brown, G. M. Coping with stress: Parallelism between the effects of septal lesions on growth hormone and corticosterone levels. *Biol. Psychiatry* 11:583–597, 1976a.

Seggie, J., and Brown, G. M. Twenty-four hour resting prolactin levels in male rats: The effect of septal lesions and order of sacrifice. *Endocrinology* 98:1516–1522, 1976b.

Stern, E., Mickey, M. R., and Gorski, R. A. Neuroendocrine factors in experimental carcinogenesis. *Ann. N.Y. Acad. Sci.* 164:494–507, 1969.

Vanhaelst, L., van Cauter, E., Degaute, J. P., and Goldstein, J. Circadian variations of serum thyrotropin levels in man. *J. Clin. Endocrinol. Metab.* 35:479–482, 1972.

Weitzman, E. D., Fukushima, D., Nogeire, C., Roffwarg, H., Gallagher, T. F., and Hellman, L. Twenty-four hour pattern of episodic secretion of cortisol in normal subjects. *J. Clin. Endocrin.* 33:14–22, 1971.

4

The Biological Axis of Senescence, Stress, and Aging as Construct for Cancer, Disease, and Death

Stacey B. Day, M.D., Ph.D., D.Sc. with the assistance of O. Garzon Duhov, Ph.D.

It is a fact that over long years of intellectual, innovative, and practical biologic research, not to mention the disbursement of vast sums of money, the experimental sciences have in the main focused their efforts on deriving an understanding of *life*. Few, if any, research studies have attempted to understand death at the molecular level. Such death presumably is the end point of all life, and in that sense is as naturally and as inextricably tied to the life process as is birth. Declining and dying are fundamental parts of the evolutionary chain including life, and clearly death is as much a process built into the biophysiologic whole as are stress, metabolism, growth, regeneration, aging, disease, and other "life" functions. The dearth of experimental studies addressed to the

Stacey B. Day • Member and Professor, Sloan-Kettering Institute for Cancer Research, New York, New York 10021. O. Garzon Duhov • Sloan-Kettering Institute for Cancer Research, New York, New York 10021.

subject of death is in marked contrast to the surfeit of writing on the moral order, for whether provoked by conscience or not, philosophic and metaphysical writings are no strangers to the bibliographical index of death studies. In recent years (Day, 1971, 1973) cultural anthropology and sociology (Calhoun, 1973) have added thrust to this dimension. The time is certainly appropriate to urge encouragement of basic research into the mechanisms of the death process. This paper discusses some aspects of the subject and reviews interacting physiologic concepts that concern potentialities for extension of life and death, as well as possibilities for actually extrapolating life to the extreme end of the survival curve. It is emphasized that this report focuses on "natural death." Provoked death" (suicides, homicides, accidental death, etc.) are not studied here. Further, without intending to arrive at an accurate all-embracing definition of death, the author's biologic working definition (Day, 1973) is stated and distinguished from that late state in time understood as senescence. The practical importance of these views can be recognized, for while few would deny the inevitability of death, most would question whether, by control of the aging process or other biologic master mechanisms (endocrine or immunologic system), it may be worthwhile postponing death, or arresting, halting, or otherwise interfering with the natural biologic mechanisms that control aging and the ultimate death act—be it volitional or involitional, in cancer, in stress, or in other disease.

If we accept a concept of death as being definable in terms of increasing entropy, then when a cell has lost all organizational power, directional flow of energy is usually halted. At the critical point in time when organization fails, the process of death may be considered to have been initiated, *the sole proviso being that the process so set in motion is irreversible.* The ability of an organism to survive (it being a total aggregate of all of its cells) is a measure of the degree to which it can free itself of excess entropy. It is this ability to so free itself that will determine the well-being of the organism, and it is this freedom which will determine life and death (Day, 1973). Senescence, on the other hand, is deterioration accompanying the passing of time, the factors responsible for its development presently being relatively poorly understood, but which if allowed to proceed unchecked *will* ultimately result in death. Precise qualitative and quantitative studies in terms of all selective cell populations still need to be done. Meanwhile, acceptance has been gained for the term *aging* to reflect a biologic chronologic passage of time conventionally synonymous with understanding implicitly recognized in degrees of senescence.

A manual and computer literature search done under the headings of "nonpsychological aspects of aging, death, and mortality" for the period 1972 through early 1974 provided 1044 references, the majority of which were reviewed in the following categories: studies of specific biological or functional changes with age; mortality studies due to some specified causes or demographic concern including cancer; a plethora of papers reviewing, classifying, and documenting present theories on aging including aspects of stress; and empirical work validating or challenging these concepts. Comfort has elsewhere (1964) reviewed many of the theories on aging since Weissman (1882). The present discussion will selectively refer to a few of the older and some of the newer theories with a viewpoint toward relating their ideological content to contemporary considerations in death research, particularly of stress- and cancer-related cell perspectives.

Human Survival

Conventionally the increasing force of mortality (i.e., decreased life expectancy) is demonstrable in a mathematical plot of the number of survivors of a given population against the age of this same group of people—in other words, study of survival curves. The primary sources for the generation of such curves are life insurance tables, and from these data a picture of senescence is also demonstrable. Probably the survival curves for various human populations as described by Comfort (1956) are most well known. However, in order to derive meaningful *scientific* conclusions, precise methodology used in constructing such tables is required and should include among other parameters details and criteria for choosing each select population sample, actual population representation in the sampling, and environmental and ecologic variables that may play a critical role in evaluating and interpreting such data. Given a family of curves such as those described by Comfort, a number of speculative conclusions have been drawn:

(1) In general, the shape of the curve is a function of the standard of living achieved by the population.
(2) In particular, improving sanitation, nutrition, and health conditions result in a shift of the age–death curve to the right— toward a rectangular type curve.
(3) The initial decline, due to infant mortality, is more severe in developing countries.
(4) The maximum life-span is approximately 90–95 years of age for all societies, and apparently has not changed much through recorded history. Conceivably, this limit could be extended to a possible maximum of 110–120 years in the future.
(5) The mean life-span or life expectancy at birth has increased over the last 20 years, reaching a plateau of about 70 years in the developed countries, and has not markedly increased since.
(6) Probability of death at an early age is rapidly decreasing.

When comparing the relative senescence of two countries, care must be taken against erroneous interpretations. For example, if Comfort's family of curves are reviewed without perception, it may seem that the population of British India for 1921–1930 was more senescent than the American population during those years. A moment of reflection will lead to the realization that these two populations were exposed to many different intrinsic and extrinsic parameters—climate, nutrition, standards of hygiene, health care and sanitation, as well as economic and sociological variations in the cultural milieus. Therefore, an uncorrected type of comparison has little real meaning. If critical conclusions are to be drawn from families of mathematically tabulated data suggesting a model for *human* mortality, then statistically controlled sampling must reflect homogeneous selections, derived from comparable demographic situations and populations of similar physical, emotional, and compensatory cultural makeup, by data analysts proficient enough to adjust the results they obtain to reflect meaningful content of information. This may not be feasible in a diversity of mobile popu-

lations, *under variant stresses and constraints,* and frequently genetically dissimilar in terms of their basic physiologic adjustments to
environment, nurture, and disease—especially cancer.

The paper of Barnes *et al.* (1974) on the *Role of Natural Consequences in the Changing Death Patterns* is of great interest. The study
was performed in Graz, Austria, where a single hospital was used
for routine hospitalization, providing an adequate cross-sectional
sampling of a population of 230,000. Complementary studies included mandatory autopsy, and diet and technological developments comparable to those in the U.S.A. Investigators arrived at
the conclusion that the eradication of tuberculosis gave rise to prolongation of life-span, allowing myocardial infarction to present as
a new "major" cause of death! Such studies as this *will* produce
meaningful data for survival curve analysis. Similarly important
are the observations of Mitra (1973) on the efficiency of estimates of
life table functions and those of Rao on long-term mortality trends
in the United States using innovative parameters for analysis of the
life tables. Thus, Rao showed that between 1900 and 1960 an increase in mortality occurred on a basis of sex and race differences.
These views lead to the not unreasonable concensus of opinion
that in order to prolong the human life-span, all underlying, non-
disease-related biophysiologic factors in senescence and its related
states must be determined, as well as such physiologic and endo-
crinologic aspects of life as are influenced by stress and neoplastic
diseases.

As early as 1825 Gompertz suggested a mathematical expression to "fit" the shape of an aging population,

$$R_n = R_0 e^{\alpha t}$$

where R_n was the mortality rate at time t, and R_0 was the rate of
birth obtained by extrapolating the exponential curve to $t = 0$. This
function does not represent the mortality at birth, for the Gompertz function is not valid during periods of growth and development. Other modifications to this function were derived by Perks
(1932), Mekeham (1867), and other statisticians. Recently Rosenberg *et al.* (1973) introduced a two-constant power law function,

$$R_n = At^n$$

where *A* is a function of temperature and is derived from the activation enthalpy for death, a value of approximately 4–5 for all species tested by these investigators. Such studies as this suggest a mathematical basis for the prediction of the human life span prolongation with a decrease in core body temperature.

Human Physiologic Responses to Aging

In general respects, the normal physiologic response to aging is reflected in a decline in most, if not all, body functions. Inevitably, interrelated changes in morphologic structure and homeostasis control occur *pari passu*, and characteristically biochemical, biological, and physiological parameters may show alterations which can be statistically correlated with chronologic aging. Such secondary effects (they are results, not causes, of aging) include eye and ear decline, changes in enzyme activity, molecular structural changes in tissues related with protein collagen, as well as chromosome alterations which via genetic information relays in the cell may result in loss of neurological, endocrinological, and immunological information (von Han, 1972). Generally speaking, there is a progressive reduction in adaptability to stress and in the capacity of the system to maintain homeostasis equilibrium characteristic of the adult at the end of growth and development (Comfort, 1968).

Aging Hypotheses

An aging–death relationship bears examination in terms of many of the hypotheses that have been put forward. Table 1 summarizes the statement of evidence on some models of aging as accepted by the Association for the Advancement of Research. In view of the remarkable structure of the human body, it would seem that only at the molecular cellular level could one reasonably expect to find a unifying concept of aging–death mechanisms. It is from a molecular-oriented basis that the goals of death-oriented research might best take shape; and with the background of presently available theories, it seems not unreasonable to feel that there is sufficient reason to proceed with empirical experiments directed to-

TABLE 1. Summary of Some Models of Aging*

Name of model	Description of model
DNA mutation or breakage	Loss of cellular synthesis due to genetic damage
Cross-linkage	Loss of cellular synthesis due to genetic damage
Inhibitor-repressor accumulation	Due to loss of message synthesis ability
Absence of adjunct factors (tRNA, rRNA, RNA polyerase)	Due to loss of message synthesis ability
Nonspecific loss of protein synthetic capacity	Loss of message translating ability
Loss of ability to translate certain messages	Codon restriction model
Mitochondrial and plastid deterioration	Loss of cellular function during age due to deterioration of semiautonomous or symbiotic organelles
Accumulation of serum factors	Inhibitory serum factors may accumulate (carrel)
Accumulation of autoantibodies	
Accumulation of symbiotic viruses	
Accumulation of exogenous precipitates	(e.g., calcium slats)
Accumulation of cross-linkages	Certain proteins, collagen, for example, become cross-linked with age
Accumulation of thermally denatured products	
Accumulation of partially hydrocysed residues	

*After Association for the Advancement of Aging Research.

ward obtaining evidence either for or against the hypotheses that have been propounded. Whether ultimate integration of these experimental findings into the biophysiologic realm is desirable to either delay, engineer, or arrest the senescence–death process is a matter for another forum than the present one. Among the most widely accepted theories at present are those derived from the concepts of age-related genetic, evolutionary, or somatic mutations. These theories are directly or indirectly related to the two currently most accepted relevant hypotheses on aging, the *clonal finitude* and *protein* hypotheses.

In 1961, Hayflick and Moorhead reported that *in vitro* normal diploid cells from human fibroblast undergo approximately 50 population doublings before entering into a phase in which growth capacity declines. They interpreted this phenomenon as a cellular manifestation of human aging. This finitude of normal diploid cells has been verified in several laboratories, convincingly putting an end to the myth of *in vitro* immortality of culture cells. In 1973, Hayflick reported additional data confirming that hypothermic storage does not affect the number of doublings. The cells act as if "remembering" in what doubling stage they were left before storage. Hayflick's original findings of an inverse relationship between donor age and culture longevity were precisely determined by Martin *et al.* (1970). The average number of divisions obtained declines by 0.20 for each year of the donor's life. Hayflick rhetorically addresses the possibility of potential immortality given to a host whose cells are continually renewed. Presently available experimental evidence appears weighted against this view (Daniel, 1971). Hayflick has pointed out that cancerous cells and germ cells escape this limitation.

Progeria and Werner's syndrome have been used as a model for aging. Patients with these diseases present characteristics and symptoms frequently found in old age. Martin *et al.* (1970) and Goldstein (1969, 1971) compared the number of cell doublings in patients with these diseases and found a marked reduction of cell proliferation *in vitro* as compared to control cultures. These results give support to Hayflick's hypothesis, although it is by no means certain that these syndromes are unqualified models for aging (Spencer and Herman, 1973). Maciera-Coelho (1966) and Litwin (1972) disputed the *in vitro* clonal finitude concept of Hayflick on the grounds that if the culture medium were to be improved, delay of senescence would follow. It may be that an increase of cell divisions is associated with changes in the chromosome and functional failure (Houck *et al.*, 1971). The number of doublings in different species appears to be related to the life-span of the species, although there is as yet no certain evidence of this.

In 1963, Orgel described the theoretical implication of error in protein synthesis, which in some cases leads to an "error catastrophe." He interpreted this accumulation of errors as a possible cause of the deterioration associated with aging. He further pointed out that in the case of germ cells, the "new and fresh start" may be attributed to some stronger selection in the growing embryo—a necessary accuracy of protein synthesis to insure successful completion of embryogenesis or other special mechanism that would decrease the frequency of errors. Similar speculation has been put forth by Medvedev and Cutler.

Orgel updated a revised hypothesis in 1973. Originally, he had thought of a diverging error frequency. He appears now to believe that it may be possible to have a protein synthetic apparatus containing a small number of errors, synthesizing another apparatus containing even fewer errors. Notwithstanding this, he cites the work of Printz (1967) and Lewis and Holliday (1970) as evidence in favor of his original theory.

Orgel's error theory encouraged a great many other studies associated with the same conceptual theme. Holliday and Tarrant (1972)—based on their experimental findings of heat-labile enzymes—integrated concepts of somatic mutations, error theory, and genetic influence. These investigators ascribed to the cytoplasm site the role of build-up error in protein synthesis. Griffiths (1973) reported that the presence of deuterium in water is the cause of a possible chemical rather than stochastic explanation for the initiation of Orgel's error catastrophe theory. Lewis (1972) pointed out that the rate of protein synthesis must be considered. He claimed that under restrictive growth conditions, as in the case of nitrogen starvation, there is an increase of error—thus indicating a relation between growth condition and prolongation of life. Although Frolkis (1973) does not acknowledge Orgel's work, his findings are in direct relation to it. Senescence is attributed to hyperpolarization of cellular membranes due to a shift in protein biosynthesis.

Wiegel and collaborators (1973), in an attempt to quantify some of the fundamental characteristic functions of Orgel's theory, introduced the concept of *vitality* in their model for aging, as well as transcription and translation parameters.

In an interesting synthesis of views, Sir MacFarlane Burnet (1973, 1974) developed a theory of an *intrinsic mutagenesis* encompassing concepts of mutations and genetic perspectives as well as an integration of the hypotheses of Hayflick and Orgel. Burnet contended that the life-span characteristic of different species is

genetically determined and developed during evolution. The concept of intrinsic mutagenesis is thought of as a bridge facilitating
information on genome and soma. Thus, the enzymes responsible
for DNA replication are the ones that play the most important role
in the genetically controlled somatic mutations. The vital role of
enzymatic surveillance is exemplified in the absence of recuperation after heavy irradiation (10,000 rads) of fibroblast cells taken
from patients with progeria. Control cells have a time recuperation
phase of half an hour (Epstein, 1973). This inadequacy of repair
mechanism is attributed to a possible missing specific enzyme. In
Burnet's view, aging is predominantly the result of somatic mutations in the line of somatic cells which continue clonal proliferation
through life. He further speculated that the indirect assessing of
somatic mutations when errors are over a certain threshold—
Orgel's error catastrophe—would ultimately be demonstrable as
the *Hayflick limit.* Burnet has suggested, based on characteristics of
the thymus—hyperactive mitoses in the cortex, inability to account
for more than a very small fraction of the cells produced, intense
liability to stress, atrophy, virtual disappearance in middle age—
that it is in this organ where the *in vivo* Hayflick limit is manifested.
However, he does not exclude other cell lines as the sites of the
Hayflick limit manifestation. His contention is that the thymus is
the first organ that reaches the Hayflick limit. New antigens produced during the time that these changes are developing and their
interaction with the population of immunocytes already present
are, in Burnet's opinion, the primary reason for the deterioration
processes common to human sensecence.

Some aspects of the empirical and theoretical evidence in support or denial of Burnet's hypothesis are:

(1) Williamson and Askonas (1973) studied in mice the senescence
    of an antibody-forming clone of cells. Burnet viewed this as
    positive evidence for his suggestion of the thymus as a "biolog-
    ical clock that allowed phenotypic expression of genetically de-
    termined age."
(2) Walford and his several associates (1969, 1973/1974) em-
    phasized the role of autoimmunity in the process of aging.
    Based on experimental studies in mice, they have attributed to

the thymus a high sensitivity to dietary restriction which may provide a deaccelerating effect on aging.

(3) Field and Shenton (1973) described a method to determine the appearance of new antigens in aging tissues. If this technique is confirmed, these investigators consider that it may provide a useful tool for comparing calendar and physiological aging and conditions which may accelerate or delay the aging process. In particular, this methodology might prove useful in the study of individuals of reputed longevity.

It should be said also, however, that Brautbar, Payne, and Hayflick (1972) discredited the immunologic theory of aging on the basis of their findings of unaltered histocompatibility antigens on normal human fibroblasts.

These hypotheses certainly must be included among those provocative views attempting to explain the deterioration mechanisms that, if unchecked, will ultimately lead to death. Broad biological studies on sleep, death-related states (catalepsy), analysis of survival curves, potential prolongation of life, and energy concepts (the dormancy of life in seeds), all contribute to possible experimental avenues for the biological study of death, as well as to interpretation of possible intermediate phases that mark the "non-death" character of cancer cells.

Increase in Life-Span

From the available literature, one infers that approaches to this chimera have been largely palliative in nature. No significant prolongation of life-span can reasonably be expected unless major changes are engineered with a view to biologically perturbing the effects of evolutionary and/or genetic sequences. As indicated above, Rosenberg (1973) has proposed a two-constant power law function to substitute for the Gompertz function. Evaluating the U.S. white mortality data for 1967, survival curves were constructed for total causes of death, specific causes of death, a theoretical curve from which major causes of death were subtracted, and survival curves for different core body temperatures. It is of remarkable interest that the curve in which the major causes of death were "eradicated" revealed a median survival time of 98.8 years and an approximate maximum life span of 130 years. With a reduction of 2°C in the core body temperature, the median survival time is 100 years, and the maximum life-span approximately 150 years. These investigators substantiated their speculation on the effect of lowering the body temperature, indicating that the organism would develop a mechanism equivalent to the one that allows the testes to be kept at a temperature of 2–8°C below the body temperature. It can be seen that in this case, where a substantial increase in the maximum life span is theoretically achieved, it is done with expectation that a certain evolutionary or genetic characteristic might evolve. Possible stress-related studies as they may (or may not) interact with such models would be informative.

Dietary Restrictions—Caloric Undernutrition

As mentioned, Walford et al. (1974) claimed a deceleration of aging through a maturation delay of the immune system. Although reducing age-associated autoimmune disease, this approach does not appear to provide a substantial change in maximum life span. Comparable conclusions appear to be derived from studies of the effects of reduction of protein error, molecular cross-links, heat-labile enzymes, lysosome enzymes, free radicals, functional decrements in postmitotic cells, etc. Reference might also be made to Comfort's work on "diagnosis of senescence" (1969) and the observation of Calloway (1974) on heat production and senescence—in which view there is a limiting value beyond which terminal senescence is seen as commencing. Finally, Eave's (1973) conjecture that the study of the "rejuvenation" process should be focused on the haploid state offers an intriguing possibility for studies on longevity. This state was chosen by Eaves because of its unique characteristics. Here the germ cells are part of the parent (premeiosis) and part of the offspring (postfertilization).

Universality of Death

Is there a universality of death? Do all species die? Unicellular organisms appear to be essentially immortal. The simplest protozoans evade death by dividing into two new organisms. Is this a type of immortality potentially reached by the germ cells? Or by cancer cells? Is the price of passage from unicellular to multicellular form aging and death? Or is it the result of sexual reproduction?

A not unrelated question for which the answer may soon be forthcoming is: "Do cells die?" Hayflick's *in vitro* experiment on the limit of cell proliferation has provided a partial answer. Should this prove to be correct for *all* cells in *all* species, *in vitro* and *in vivo*, the statement of "normality" of cell death might hold true—although the body, as we conventionally view it, is a macroatomic macrocellular structure in which even in "death" some cells are turning over in biologically "life" phases. In the case of nondividing cells, they may be maintained *in vitro* a certain length of time depending on the species from which they were obtained. As senescence starts, functional decrements begin. It is conceivable that the recently published studies of Veomett *et al.* (1974)—on reconstruction of mammalian cells from nuclear and cytoplasmic components—might provide a useful tool to evaluate many aspects of Hayflick's hypotheses.

Clearly, senescence and death are related. If death is ultimately thought of as an evolutionary mode to improve the species, and generation a tool to selectively improve it, then one might concede a parallel between death as an intrinsic part of morphogenesis created with a view to eliminate effete or obsolete organs and the absolute death of higher animals. It is not unreasonable to derive a correlation from this view in an effort to account for the difference in life span between different species and among the same species for other variables (i.e., sex and race).

Summary Conclusions

Based upon the large number of publications reviewed, and emphasizing the relatively few *experimental* investigations on the biology of death, we may conclude that intellectual studies heretofore have been concerned in the main with exploring the feasibility of a postponement of death, and with cultural and social evaluation of the attitudes of individuals and societies to death and dying. The second proposition is not properly within the scope of this paper. In respect to prolongation of life, aging, the role of stress, postponement of death, and death, such studies as are available would seem to suggest that genetic manipulation appears at this time to promise both qualitatively and quantitatively the best success of achieving a substantial improvement in aging and a postponement of death. Moreover, paradoxically, if a delay of the end of life is to be achieved, the beginning of it should be more closely scrutinized. With current sophisticated biochemical methodologies, experimental techniques involving determination of the karyoplast structure in the germ cell might produce evidence concerning such issues as the existence of reiterative genes, their number, the minimal number required for a "fresh start" in the embryo, the nature and description of artificial mutations, etc.

Study of hybrid cells formed from early embryos or from premeiosis cells and somatic cells might provide scientific bases for the feasibility and potentiality of genetic manipulation and evidence for the "rejuvenation" stage between meiosis and fertilization. It is suggested that it is in these and similar schemes that aging and death might reasonably be scientifically evaluated in future investigative studies.

References

Barnes, B. O., Ratzenhofer, M., and Gisi, R. The role of natural consequences in the changing death patterns. *J. Am. Geriatr. Soc.*22:176, 1974.

Burnet, M. F. An immunological approach to aging. *Lancet* August 15:358–360, 1970.

Burnet, M. F. Aging and immunological surveillance. *Triangle*2:159–162, 1973.

Burnet, M. F. Intrinsic mutagenesis: A genetic basis of aging. *Pathology*6:1, 1974.

Brautbar, C., Payne, R., and Hayflick, L. Fate of HL-A in aging cultured human diploid cell strains. *Exp. Cell Res.*75:31, 1972.

Calhoun, J. B. Death squared: The explosive growth and demise of a mouse population. *Proc. Roy. Soc. Med.*66:80–88, 1973.

Calloway, N. O. Heat production and senescence. *J. Am. Geriatr. Soc.*22:149, 1974.

Comfort, A. *Aging: The Biology of Senescence.* London: Routledge & Kegan Paul, 1964.

Comfort, A. Feasibility in age research. *Nature*217:320, 1968.

Comfort, A. Test battery to measure aging–rate in man. *Lancet* December 27:1411, 1969.

Cutler, R. G. Redundancy of information content in the genome of mammalian species as a protective mechanism determining aging rate. *Mech. Aging Dev.*2:381, 1973/74.

Daniel, C. W., Young, L. J. T., Medina, D., and DeOme, K. B. The influence of mammogenic hormones on serially transplanted mouse mammary gland. *Exp. Gerontol.*6:95, 1971.

Day, S. B. *Death and Attitudes towards Death.* Minneapolis: Bell Museum of Pathobiology, University of Minnesota Medical School, 1972.

Day, S. B. *Tuluak and Amaulik. Dialogues on Death and Mourning with the Innuit Eskimo of Point Barrow and Wainwright, Alaska.* Minneapolis: Bell Museum of Pathobiology, University of Minnesota Medical School, 1973.

Day, S. B. Death: Failure to direct energy flow and an expression of disorganization at the molecular level. In: R. A. Good, S. B. Day, and J. Yunis (Eds.), *Molecular Pathology.* Springfield, Ill.: Charles C Thomas, 1975.

Eaves, G. A. Consequence of normal diploid cell mortality. *Mech. Aging Dev.*2:19, 1973.

Epstein, J., Williams, J. R., and Little, J. B. Deficient DNA repair in human progeroid cells. *Proc. Nat. Acad. Sci. USA.*70:977, 1973.

Field, E. J., and Shenton, B. K. Emergence of new antigens in aging tissues. *Gerontologia*19:211, 1973.

Frolkis, V. V. Functions of cells and biosynthesis of protein in aging. *Gerontologia*19:189, 1973.

Goldstein, S. Life span of cultured cells in progeria. In *Letters to the Editor. Lancet*1:424, 1969. February 22, 1969.

Gompertz, B. On the nature of the function expressive of the law of human mortality and on a new mode of determining life contingencies. *Phil. Trans. R. Soc. (London), Series A*115:513, 1825.

Griffiths, T. R. A new unifying theory for the initiation of aging mechanisms and processes. *Mech. Aging Dev.*2:295, 1973.

Hayflick, L. The longevity of cultured human cells. *J. Am. Geriatr. Soc.*22:1–12, 1974.

Hayflick, L. The limited in vitro lifetime of human diploid cell strains. *Exp. Cell Res.*37:614–636, 1965.

Hayflick, L., and Moorhead, B. S. The serial cultivation of human diploid cell strain. *Exp. Cell Res.*25:582, 1961.

Holliday, R., and Tarrant, G. M. Altered enzymes in aging human fibroblasts. *Nature*238:26–30, 1972.

Houck, J. C., Sharma, V. K., and Hayflick, L. Functional failures of cultured human diploid fibroblast after continued population doublings. *Proc. Soc. Exp. Biol. Med.*137:331–333, 1971.

Lewis, C. M. Protein turnover in relation to Orgel's error theory of aging. *Mech. Aging Dev.*1:43–47, 1972.

Litwin, J. Human diploid cell response to variations in relative amino acid concentration in eagle medim. *Exp. Cell. Res.*72:566–568, 1972.

Maciera-Coelho, A. Action of cortisone on human fibroblast *in vitro. Experientia.* 22:390–I, 1966.

Martin, G. M., Sprague, C. A., and Epstein, C. J. Replicative life-span of cultivated human cells. *Lab. Invest.*23:86–92, 1970.

Medvedev, Z. A. Repetition of molecular genetic as a possible factor in evolutionary changes of life-span. *Exp. Gerontol.*7:227, 1972.

Mekeham,W. M. On the law of mortality. *J. Inst. Actu.*13:325, 1867.

Mitra, S. On the efficiency of the estimates of life table functions. *Demography*10: 421, 1973.

Orgel, L. E. The maintenance of the accuracy of protein synthesis and its relevance to aging. *Biochemistry*49:517–521, 1963.

Orgel, L. E. Aging of clones of Mammalian Cells. *Nature*243:441–445, 1973.

Perks, W. On some experiments in the graduation of mortality statistic. *J. Inst. Actu.*63:12, 1932.

Printz, D. B., and Gross, S. R. An apparent relationship between mistranslation and an altered leucyl–TRNA synthetase in a conditional lethal mutant of *Neurospora crassa*. *Genetics*55:451, 1967.

Rao, S. L. N. On long-term mortality trends in the United States, 1850–1968. *Demography*10:405, 1973.

Rosenberg, B., Kemeny, G., Smith, L. G., Skurnick, I. D., and Bandurski, M. J. The kinetics and thermodynamics of death in multicellular organisms. *Mech. Aging Dev.*1–2:275–293, 1973.

Spence, A. M., and Herman, M. M. Critical re-examination of the premature aging concept in Progeria: A light and exectron microscopic study. *Mech. Aging Dev.* 2:211–217, 1973.

Veomett, G. Prescott, D. M., Shay, J., and Porter, K. R. Reconstruction of mammalian cells from nuclear and cytoplasmic components separated by treatment with Cytocholasin B. *Proc. Nat. Acad. Sci. USA*71:1999, 1974.

Von Hahn, H. P. Primary causes of aging: A brief review of some modern theories and concepts. *Mech. Aging Dev.*2:245–250, 1973.

Walford, R. L., Liu, R. K., Gerbase-Delima, M., Mathies, M., and Smith, G. S. Long-term dietary restriction and immune function in mice: Response to sheep red blood cells and to mitogenic agent. *Mech. Aging Dev.*2:447–454, 1973/74.

Walford, R. L. *The Immunologic Theory of Aging*. Baltimore: Williams and Wilkins, 1969.

Weismann, A. *The Germ Plasm: A Theory of Heredity*. (Translated by W. N. Parker.) London: Walter Scott, 1893.

Weismann, A. *The Duration of Life. Essays upon Heredity and Kindred Biological Problems*. (Authorized translation from the German. E. D. Poulton, Ed.) Oxford: Oxford Clarendon Press, 1889.

Wiegel, D., Beier, W., and Brehme, Karl-Heinz. Vitality and error rate in biological systems: Some theoretical considerations. *Mech. Aging & Dev.*2:117, 1973.

Williamson, A. R., and Askonas, B. A. Senescence of an antibody forming cell clone. *Nature*238:337–339, 1972.

5

Advanced Malignant Disease and the Person Under Stress

Balfour Mount, M.D., F.R.C.S.(C)

The Patient, the Family, and the Care Giver

A 1973 study at Royal Victoria Hospital in Montreal made it clear that the hospital was seriously deficient in meeting the needs of its terminally ill patients and their families.[1] In striking contrast, it appeared that St. Christopher's Hospice, London, England was effectively decreasing the stress experienced by patients with terminal disease, their families, and the medical team caring for them.

The 1973 study indicated the patients' desire for complete openness and honesty in discussions of diagnosis and prognosis, the physician's reluctance to be that candid, the resident's relative lack of concern for the patient's emotional needs and the social worker's tendency to minimize the problem. It became evident that the acute treatment ward was an inappropriate setting for patients with terminal disease, heightening the stress of all concerned. The study also suggested that when treatment designed at modifying the natural history of the disease is no longer appropriate, patients experience increasing isolation. The medical team make less fre-

Balfour Mount • Director, Palliative Care Unit, Royal Victoria Hospital, McGill University, Montreal, Quebec, H3A 1A1, Canada.

quent visits. The patients' deteriorating medical status is emphasized by the improvement in the condition of neighboring acute care patients. Families are quick to notice these contrasts and their anxieties are thus exacerbated. The situation is also unpleasant for other acute care patients for whom the presence of a terminally ill neighbor is frequently anxiety-producing.

The 1973 study also suggested that members of the medical team who recognized the serious deficiencies in the care of the terminally ill frequently felt impotent, guilty, and angry at the system that makes more appropriate care impossible. What was equally striking was the frequency with which the medical team was completely oblivious to serious patient and family stress. Members of the health care team tended to see themselves as being personally more sensitive to the needs of these patients than their colleagues are. A further finding of interest was that the physician's attitude toward his own death appeared to be a determinant in establishing how he perceived his patient's needs. The irrelevance of the hard-won skills of the general hospital at investigating, diagnosing, prolonging life, and curing was seen as an important variable leading to the isolation these patients and their families experience. [2]

The recommendation that a hospice unit or "palliative care unit" be established at Royal Victoria Hospital to explore the possibility of providing care similar to that provided at St. Christopher's Hospice—but within a general hospital setting—was a natural outcome of the research data compiled.

The Palliative Care Service is comprised of four major functions: The Palliative Care Unit itself, the Home Care Program, the Consultation Team, and a Bereavement Follow-up Group. Evaluation of the impact of this service indicates that it is effective in reducing the stress experienced by terminally ill patients and their families. [3,4] The emphasis is on the quality of life rather than death. The multidisciplinary team is concerned with the needs of both patient and family—psychological, spiritual, financial, and interpersonal, as well as medical. With the provision of specialized nursing care, expertise in the management of pain and other symptoms, the assurance of continuity in care, and a bed without a parking meter on it, the experience of the patient–family units involved has usually been transformed from one characterized by out-of-control symptoms, anxiety, and strained relationships to one of symptom control and reconciliation.

While the stress experienced by the Palliative Care team has been significant, the professional gratification has been great and the staff turnover no higher than on other services. The emotional cost involved in this type of crisis intervention is significant. In the initial months of the pilot project, the staff stress was extremely high. The stress of a pioneering endeavor, confrontations with the traditional medical care model, the demanding complexities of the problems encountered, and the recurring reminders of man's mortality were seen as important factors in escalating staff stress. [5]

The service policy of encouraging the recognition and expression of emotions adds to the common awareness of individual personal problems among staff members and this also carries a cost in terms of shared stress. A final factor comprises the highly idealistic aims and high level of motivation of the staff involved in this work.

The exceedingly high staff stress levels experienced in the first years of the pilot project have since dissipated, but staff stress remains an issue of central importance in this type of work. [5,6] Recognition of this is of great importance to those involved in the nearly 100 North American centers currently establishing units modeled after St. Christopher's Hospice and the Royal Victoria Hospital Palliative Care Unit. A careful evaluation of the stress in existing units should assist in providing useful recommendations in this quickly growing new specialty in the health care system. The emphasis on the team approach, a relaxation of formalities, the use of frequent small group discussions, the assistance of a psychiatrist whose first priority is staff stress, the presence of children, and the celebration of "life events" have been utilized in attempts to diminish the stress experienced. The crucial factors in the amelioration of staff stress, however, are the satisfaction of reducing human suffering and the opportunity of developing a deeper personal and professional philosophy toward living and dying. The staff is able to see the Palliative Care Service as a monument, not to the incurability of some pathologic processes, but to the dignity of man.

Some specific aspects of our work are now discussed:

Palliative Care of the Terminal Cancer Patient

There are only three admissible goals in the treatment of malignant disease: to cure, to prolong life, and to improve the quality of survival. In recent decades, interest and financial resources have been focused on improving the effectiveness of our skills in investigating, diagnosing, curing, and prolonging survival. Although a high percentage of oncology patients will die due to their carcinomas, little effort has gone into improving our skill in treating patients with advanced disease. There is growing evidence that these patients and their families experience a wide variety of critical problems that usually go unrecognized by those responsible for their care. The terminally ill patient, instead of receiving sympathetic understanding and expertise in meeting his medical and emotional needs, may encounter isolation and depersonalization. [2,7,8,9]

Hinton has commented "We emerge deserving of little credit; we who are capable of ignoring the conditions which make muted people suffer. The dissatisfied dead cannot noise abroad the negligence they have experienced." [10]

Defining Appropriate Therapy

The current tendency to equate excellence of medical care with aggressive investigation and therapy is a natural product of the recent rapid expansion of medical knowledge. The result is a generation of physicians conditioned to see their role exclusively as "employed by the patient to fight for his life." [11] Failure to recognize that further investigation and active treatment may be inappropriate in the presence of advanced disease has resulted in frequent unnecessary suffering. We have too often failed to recognize that the capacity to act does not, in itself, justify the action.

While therapy to prolong life is still appropriate, unproven therapeutic modalities are justifiable only as part of carefully designed and supervised clinical trials. Accepted forms of treatment may be justified only after a consideration of attendant morbidity, probability of response, and mean duration of response, in consultation with the patient and family.

When only palliative care is applicable, further investigations can be justified only if they lead directly to an increased ability to improve the quality of survival through their facilitation of improved symptom control. Investigations for research purposes are justifiable in this setting only when informed consent has been obtained from the patient.

The decision that therapy should be restricted to palliative care is made more easily if the physician's perception of his mandate embraces the broader concept of alleviating suffering rather than simply "fighting for life," and if he recognizes that the treater's need to treat and the family's need to treat are unacceptable rationales for further therapy. Such a decision should be associated with a positive statement that while therapy can no longer be expected to make an impact on the disease process, much can be done to control symptoms and assist the patient in living in homeostasis with his tumor. It may be helpful to remind all concerned that many medical problems—diabetes, arteriosclerotic vascular disease, multiple sclerosis, etc.—cannot be cured: but we can learn to live as fully as possible within the situation. The patient and family are left with the concept of an appropriate shifting in therapeutic goals by a physician who remains interested and actively involved. The statement "nothing more can be done" reflects a tragic ignorance of the complex multidimensional needs of these patients and their families and the creative therapeutic responses to these needs that are now possible.

The Nature of the Need

Our traditional preoccupation with pathophysiology as the only opportune focus of our attention is woefully inadequate in the arena of advanced disease. While the medical needs may be undeniably complex and of central concern, to them are added the complicating factors of serious psychological stress for the patient and family, strained interpersonal relationships, serious financial problems, and a cloak of ever-present metaphysical questions which these patient-family units are forced to face. "Why me? Why this suffering? Why is this allowed? Is this all there is?" Experience suggests that intervention must be directed at all these levels—physical, psychological, spiritual, social, and interpersonal if suffering is to be successfully alleviated.

Chronic Pain: Its Nature and Management

When intractable pain is present, its treatment stands as the central problem in the palliative care of patients with advanced malignant disease.

Aims of Treatment

The goals of the therapist should be:

Identify the Etiology.   Clarification of the cause is an essential first step in pain control, since it may lead to specific therapy such as focal irradiation for a bony metastasis, extraction of a carious tooth, or purgatives for pain due to constipation.

Preventing Pain.   The aim is to anticipate and forestall pain rather than merely treat it after it occurs. This requires the regular administration of appropriate amounts of analgesics, specifically titrated to the patient's current needs. There is no place for "p.r.n." medication orders as the basis of treatment of chronic pain, since the pain will repeatedly be out of control. Unnecessary suffering and escalations in analgesic dose result.

Erasing Pain Memory.   As the anxious anticipation and memory of pain is lessened by successful pain prevention, the dose of analgesic required will frequently decrease.

An Unclouded Sensorium.   Many patients feel trapped between perpetual pain on the one hand and perpetual somnolence on the other. The balance, a pain-free state without sedation, requires careful individual regulation of analgesic dose according to the patient's needs.

A Normal Affect.   The ability of a patient to relate to his environment will be enhanced by a normal affect neither euphoric nor depressed.

Ease of Administration. Oral administration of analgesics can allow a patient to retain a degree of independence and mobility that is impossible when analgesics are given parenterally. Cachexia may also make regular parenteral medication difficult and painful.

The Nature of Chronic Pain

For optimal results, the physician must recognize the important difference between *acute* and *chronic* pain. Acute pain has a beginning and an end. It may be classified as mild, moderate, or severe, and has a meaning in that it draws attention to an offending member so that corrective therapy may be applied. Chronic pain, however, can be characterized as a vicious cycle with no set time limit. The fearful anticipation of its perpetuation leads to anxiety, depression, and insomnia, which in turn accentuate the physical components of the pain. [12] Leshan suggests that meaninglessness, helplessness, and hopelessness are characteristic of the unreal nightmare world in which the patient with chronic pain lives. [13] Saunders has coined the term "total pain" to describe the all-consuming nature of chronic pain and our need to attack all if its facets—physical, psychological, spiritual, financial, and social. [14] For the patient with advanced malignant disease, pain implacably reminds him of his dismal prognosis and thus further aggravates his utter agony.

The Management of Chronic Pain

If the pain is localized, radiation therapy, nerve block, or some form of neurosurgical procedure may provide excellent control.

With moderate to severe chronic pain, only the narcotic analgesics provide adequate control. Milder analgesics should always be tried for less severe pain and may be helpful in combination with more potent drugs. A wide variety of agents is available; Catalano presents a good recent review. [15]

In the past, the use of narcotics has widely been considered "bad management." Recent studies have demonstrated, however, that all the above treatment goals may be obtained using oral narcotics without the danger of tolerance and attendant dose escalation. An oral narcotic mixture containing morphine taken in conjunction with a phenothazine provided excellent pain control in 75–80% of patients with intractable cancer pain in general hospital accommodations and in 90% of patients in a special "palliative care unit" designed to meet the needs of the terminally ill and their families. [3]

The standard mixture is a liquid containing a variable amount of morphine, 10 mg of cocaine, 2.5 ml of ethyl alcohol (98%), 5 ml of flavoring syrup, and a variable amount of chloroform water for a total of 20 ml per dose. The mixture is given regularly, every 4 hours around the clock in conjunction with a phenothiazine syrup (usually prochlorperazine starting at 5 mg, while in restless patients chlorpromazine at 10 mg may be used).

Lengthy anticipated patient survival is not a contraindication to narcotic use with careful dosage adjustment; furthermore, the mixture can be used for periods up to several years without dose escalation.

For most patients, pain relief can be obtained with 5–10 mg of morphine per dose, while in small or elderly patients as little as 2.5 mg may be effective. A pain-free state can be achieved in most patients by giving sequential increments in the narcotic dose. The usual sequential doses of morphine given in the mixture are 2.5, 5, 10, 15, 20, 30, 40, 60, 90, and 120 mg. For excrutiating pain, an alternative method is to start with a relatively high narcotic dose, subsequently adjusting the dose in sequential decrements until analgesia without sedation is achieved. Dose alteration should be made at intervals of 48–72 hours. Since narcotics and the phenothiazines are synergistic, the dose of only one variable—the narcotic or the phenothiazine—should be changed at a time. Even small dose alterations may lead to profound changes in analgesia and sedation.

It is important to reassure both patient and family that the initial drowsiness associated with the introduction of narcotics is temporary, lasting only 48–72 hours. The physician's confident reassurance that pain can be controlled undoubtedly has a beneficial effect in promoting analgesia.

Dispensing the morphine mixture and the phenothiazine syrup separately allows greater flexibility in adjusting dosage.

Once a continuous pain-free state is achieved, they may be combined in dispensing for greater ease of administration.

Careful observation of the patient's condition over a complete 24-hour period may suggest augmentation of one or two specific doses at periods of peak activity.

If parenteral medication becomes necessary, the equivalent dose of morphine is one-half the previous oral dose. Thus, a patient whose pain has been controlled with 30 mg of morphine taken orally would require 15 mg intramuscularly. [16]

Adverse Effects

Adverse effects are infrequent with this approach. Those to be watched for include sedation, nausea and vomiting, constipation, respiratory depression, tolerance–dependence, and extrapyramidal effects. The potentiation of the narcotic sedation effect by the phenothiazine has been referred to earlier. After the initial 72 hours, sustained sedation suggests that the narcotic dose is excessive. However, patients with advanced malignant disease often have other causes for somnolence, such as hapatic or renal insufficiency or intracranial metastases.

Nausea and vomiting, a common side effect of narcotics, is countered by the routine use of phenothiazines. If a patient is vomiting before therapy is instituted, control should first be achieved with parenteral medications prior to switching to the oral route.

The combined effect of poor dietary intake, dehydration, inactivity, and narcotic therapy almost invariably leads to constipation. This should be prevented by using a combination of a stool softener and a bowel stimulant such as dioctyl sodium sulfosuccinate and Senna concentrate. Clinically significant respiratory depression and tolerance with associated dose escalation are not seen when the dose has been carefully titrated to the patient's need. Marks and Sachar have commented "the excessive and unrealistic concern about the danger of addiction in the hospitalized medical patient is a significant and potent force for undertreatment with narcotic."[17] It would seem that undertreatment with analgesic medication may encourage craving and psychological dependence.

Our own experience[3] confirms that of Twycross[18] that a change in dosage requirement heralds a change in disease status rather than tolerance.

Extrapyramidal effects, orthostatic hypotension, and other side effects of the phenothiazines must be watched for, but they occur infrequently with suggested doses.

Recent experience with the use of morphine in conjunction with the phenothiazine but without the other additives of the mixture has suggested that this simplified approach is equally effective in pain control.

Careful assessment of the patient's psychological status leading to the judicious use of trycyclic antidepressants and the benzodiazepines is indicated; the additional use of antiinflammatory agents, such as phenylbutazone corticosteroids and hypnotics, may all be useful adjuncts in attacking the vicious cycle of chronic pain. The presence of a positive supportive environment is seen as a further factor in decreasing pain and assisting in its control. [3,12]

Control of Physical Symptoms Other than Pain

Attention to detail is the basis for excellence in palliative care. At this time of shifting symptom complexes and diminishing resources, frequent brief interviews with the patient for the purpose of reevaluating his status and carefully titrating his symptomatic control will pay rich dividends in averting potentially serious problems and hospitalization. The implied message—that the physician has a continuing interest in the patient's welfare—is a reassuring factor of major importance to both patient and family.

Optimum symptomatic control depends on excellence of nursing care. Again, attention to detail is important. A physician's visit will be remembered as being longer in duration and of greater meaning if the physician sits down at the bedside so that there is eye contact on the same level. How often we repeatedly look down on our patients! Touching the patient, in general, brings with it reassurance. However, it may represent an intrusion of privacy to a few. It requires sensitivity to meet the patients where they are, rather than where we feel they should be.

Of particular note is the significant experience of Saunders[14] in the symptomatic medical management of malignant bowel obstruction. She has observed that the obstruction is usually temporary, and that with time most obstructions will open up to allow passage of flatus and stool. Of further importance is her observation that vomiting is well tolerated in the absence of nausea. Malignant bowel obstruction may thus be managed with careful mouth care to control thirst, coupled with oral intake as desired, careful titration of medications to control nausea until the obstruction is relieved, and reassurance to minimize the psychological trauma of vomiting. Lomotil® (diphenoxylate hydrochloride plus atropine) tabs 2 g.i.d. may be used to control painful colic. The frequency of vomiting will depend on the level of the bowel obstruction. In the great majority of cases, bowel obstruction can be managed in these patients for prolonged periods of time (up to 26 days in the author's personal experience) with excellent patient comfort, without resorting to colostomy, nasogastric suction, or intravenous fluids. [19]

In the presence of terminal disease, a standing order for hyoscine 0.4 to 0.6 mg, to be given IM p.r.n. with morphine is a great assistance in controlling the anxiety-producing noisy terminal respirations or "death rattle" which is so distressing to relatives (if not to the patient) during the waning hours of life. This combination is also of great use in relieving distress in a major crisis such as with hemorrhage or following a pulmonary embolus. Drugs given in this setting are for the control of symptoms only. This differs significantly from the intentional prescribing of drugs with the intent of shortening life. If their use leads to an insignificant abbreviation of life, this is considered an accepted risk, taken in the interest of alleviating suffering. A clear understanding of goals will alleviate anxiety on the part of nursing staff in this situation.

Mental Distress in the Setting of Terminal Illness and Its Management

North American Indians tell us that "to understand my brother, I must walk in his moccasins." In most cases, we are at a significant disadvantage as we attempt to help the patient with advanced cancer. We may know something of the adaptations to stress he has had to make since the original diagnosis, but we frequently know little of the factors which modify those responses, his family relationships, his work, his financial concerns, his ambitions and dreams, his lifetime of experiences, achievements, failures, stresses, compensations, and struggles. In this setting, it is a help to have some understanding of our patient's fears and hopes.

The terminal patient is nearly always either consciously or unconsciously aware that death is close.[7] Kübler-Ross has suggested that there is a series of mental adjustments which we may go through in coming to terms with the fact we have a serious or life-threatening disease. These include denial, anger, bargaining, depression, and finally acquiescence. Whatever the sequence in a given patient, one can usually find a subtle balance between a realistic acceptance on the one hand and simultaneous rejection on the other. In dying, we are challenged to adapt, not to a single loss, but rather to a series of losses: job, mobility, strength, physical and mental capacity, and plans for the future.

It is helpful to recognize that the patient's family will go through a similar series of mental adjustments. An understanding of this process will assist the physician in gracefully accepting the anger of the patient or relatives when it is directed at him and in mediating more skillfully when it is directed at the family member involved.

References

1. Mount, B. M., Jones, A., and Patterson, A. Death and dying: Attitudes in a teaching hospital. *Urology*4:741, 1974.
2. Mount, B. M. The problem of caring for the dying in a general hospital; the palliative care unit as a possible solution. *CMAJ*115:119, 1976.
3. Melzack, R., Ofiesh, J. G., and Mount, B. M. The Brompton mixture: Effects on pain in cancer patients. *CMAJ*115:125, 1976.
4. Mount, B. M. *Report of Pilot Project (January 1975–January 1977)*. Montreal: Palliative Care Service, Royal Victoria Hospital, 1976, p. 137.
5. Beszterczey, A. Staff stress on a newly developed palliative care service: The psychiatrist's role. *Can. Psychiatr. Assoc. J.*22:347, 1977.
6. Vachon, M.L.S., Lyall, W. A. L., and Freeman, S. J. J. Measurement and management of stress in health professionals working with advanced cancer patients. *Death Education:* Winter, 1978.

7. Kübler-Ross, E. *On Death and Dying.* New York: Macmillan, 1969.
8. Lasagna, L. Physicians' Behaviour Toward the Dying Patient, *The Dying Patient,* Brim, O. G., Freeman, H. E., Levine, S., and Scotch, N. (Eds.) New York: Russell Sage, 1970.
9. Duff, R. S., and Hollingshead, A. B. Dying and death. *Sickness and Society.* New York: Harper & Row, 1968.
10. Hinton, J. *Dying,* 2nd Ed. Harmondsworth, England Penguin, 159, 1972.
11. Epstein, F. H. The role of the physician in the prolongation of life. In Ingelfinger, F. J., Ebert, R. V., Finland, M., Relman, A. S. (Eds.), *Controversy in Internal Medicine.* Philadelphia: W. B. Saunders, 1974.
12. Melzack, R. *The Puzzle of Pain.* Harmondsworth, England: Penguin, 1973, p. 142.
13. Leshan, L. The world of the patient in severe pain of long duration. *J. Chronic Disease* 17:119, 1964.
14. Saunders, C. The management of terminal illness. *London Hosp. Med. Publ.,* 1967.
15. Catalano, R. Medical management of pain caused by cancer. *Semin. Oncol.* 2:378, 1975.
16. Mount, B. M., Ajemian, I., and Scott, J. F. Use of the Brompton mixture in treating the chronic pain of malignant disease. *CMAJ:*115,122, 1976.
17. Marks, M. D., and Sachar, E. J. Undertreatment of medical in-patients with narcotic analgesics. *Ann. Intern Intern Med.*78:173, 1973.
18. Twycross, R. Clinical experience with diamorphine in advanced malignant disease, *Int. J. Clin. Pharmacol.*9:184, 1974.
19. Mount, B. M. Palliative care of the terminally ill. Presented at the annual meeting of The Royal College of Physicians and Surgeons of Canada, Vancouver, British Columbia, January 27, 1978. *Ann. Royal Coll. Physicians and Surgeons of Canada,* July, 1978.

6

The Homeostatic Significance of the Death–Life Cycle Dynamics in Mental Functions

Wolfgang Luthe, M.D.

Abstract*

How do self-regulatory brain mechanisms handle the issue of death? We here limit our discussion to the data which concern the death of oneself, distinguishing between the dynamics of death as a personal issue and the complementary mental dynamics involving the death of others.

S. Freud and others based their psychoanalytic views and hypotheses about death on dreams. My observations are obtained from tape-recorded autogenic abreactions (AA) during which the subject is fully awake when undergoing AA.

After an initial 1- to 2-minute practice of the first autogenic standard exercise (i.e., heaviness formulas), the subject mentally

*This is an abstract of Dr. Luthe's detailed presentation at the symposium on Cancer, Stress, and Death held at the International Institute of Stress, Montreal, Quebec, Canada in 1977.

Wolfgang Luthe • Scientific Director, Oskar Vogt Institute and Visiting Professor, Kyūshū University, Fukuoka, Japan. Mailing address: Medical Centre, 5300 Côte des Neiges, Montreal, Québec, H3T 1Y3, Canada.

shifts to the passive acceptance (P.A.) stage of the autogenic state. Then he begins to describe the complex dynamics of successively unfolding mental elaborations (e.g., sensory, visual, olfactory, vestibular, motor, ideational). These prohomeostatic elaborations are programmed by unknown mechanisms, yet follow observable patterns in a self-regulatory fashion. Observing the principle of noninterference, the subject delegates all tasks of programming to relevant brain mechanisms (i.e., as in dreams). He remains a passively accepting observer, as if watching and describing a television program.

The brain-directed elaborations during the P.A.-stage of the autogenic state are in many respects similar to dreams. However, they are dynamically more coherent, sequentially better organized, and convey a "clearer script" of content. They are more efficient than dreams in producing prohomeostatic adjustments.

Observations from autogenic abreactions show patterns that are compatible with the Freudian distinction of the two primal instincts of life (*Eros*) and death (*Thanatos*). Freudian views emphasize the destructive aspects of the death instinct and its energy (*destrudo*). The self-regulatory brain functions during AA consistently convey that the mental dynamics released by, for example, viewing one's own death in cinerama fashion are basically highly constructive, liberating, and clearly prohomeostatic.

The self-regulatory brain dynamics observed in subjects experiencing AA also provided new information about the psychodynamic and homeostatic significance of events that are related to one's own death. Already considered by S. Freud were such variables as aggression, self-punishment, death-wishes, and fear of birth (birth trauma). We find through AA that a variety of accidents and traumas also play a prominent role: traffic and sports accidents, artificial alterations of consciousness (e.g., intoxications, suffocation, fainting), injuries (particularly to the cranial region), extensive bleeding, and certain medical procedures (e.g., inhalation anesthesia, ECT). Death dynamics are stimulated and reinforced by identification with others (e.g., death of close persons, Christ, TV heroes, accident victims). Furthermore, self-regulatory brain elaborations consistently showed that anxiety-promoting forms of religious education are severely brain-disturbing and closely related to the dynamics of death. This is particularly so when the "second death"—burning in the eternal flames of Hell—supersedes the fear and anxiety of the "first death"—i.e., the phyical death.

Natural brain functions are given ample opportunity during AA to follow their own prohomeostatic program. This program neutralizes brain-disturbing material related to the topic of death; a variety of psychophysiologic manifestations indicate progressive revitalization. Inversely, when such natural processes of pro-homeostatic neutralization of death are not allowed, actively blocked, or avoided, there is a relatively rapid increase of tension, anxiety, and depressive manifestations. Functionally related psychophysiologic reactions are amplified. Deterioration of well-being is evident.

These findings suggest two hypotheses of interest. First, in-adequate self-regulatory neutralization of mental dynamics related to death—particularly one's own death—constitute a source of psychophysiologic stress that promotes deterioration of health (or existing disease). Secondly, ample opportunity for permitting natural brain mechanisms to freely and adequately neutralize brain-disturbing material involving the topic of death is one of the treatment modalities that helps to maintain more favorable levels of prohomeostatic self-regulation and better health.

Reference

Luthe, W. *Autogenic Therapy*, Vols. V and VI. New York: Grune & Stratton, 1970, 1973.

7

The Cancer Patient as Educator and Counselor

Barbara G. Cox, B.S.

Traditionally, the cancer patient has been a passive recipient of various therapies—exerting very little personal direction over either the management or the outcome of his or her disease. Unlike patients with diabetes or hypertension, [1] for example, cancer patients generally adopt a passive role in their treatment, aside from the actual consent to therapy or refusal thereof. The cancer patient literally presents his or her body to the clinic or hospital, where it is examined by a variety of specialists, subjected to surgery, irradiated, and/or treated with toxic chemotherapeutic agents. Through all of this, the patient often feels like an object, while the family stands by, feeling uninformed and helpless, unable to assist the patient through the various discomforts and fears he or she faces.

Barbara G. Cox • Executive Editor and Manager, Biomedical Publications, Ross Laboratories, Columbus, Ohio 43216. The work described in this chapter was done while the author was Associate Director, Cancer Rehabilitation Program, Mayo Comprehensive Cancer Center. It was funded by Contract CN 45120 from the National Cancer Institute.

The Emergence of Self-Help Groups

Increasingly, however, patients and their families have begun to assert themselves on the health care scene, declaring their need for information and support. [2] This has become evident through the self-help groups that have sprung up in recent years. The American Cancer Society was among the initiators of such programs. For example, *Reach to Recovery* volunteers (women who have successfully undergone mastectomy) visit other women with mastectomies postoperatively to give them support, encouragement, and rehabilitation training. [3,4] *Ostomy Visitor* programs have also emerged from the American Cancer Society. [4,5] In these, a recovered ostomate visits a newly operated-upon ostomate in the hospital, giving this person not only helpful information but also visual proof that it is possible to recover from ostomy surgery and lead a normal life. *Make Today Count* is another, more recent organization of cancer patients, with chapters throughout the United States. [6] This growing coalition of cancer patients holds regular chapter meetings, enabling its members to support one another and to enjoy life one day at a time. *Candlelighters* is a nationwide network of the parents of children with cancer, who come together to offer help, encouragement, and support to each other throughout their children's disease, as well as to offer comfort if the child dies. [7]

There are many other such organizations. And their numbers grow monthly. As they come into public view, their membership climbs. Through sharing of information and learning more about the kinds of cancer they face, patients and their families are enabled to gain some sense of mastery over the disease. Knowledge is strength. Moreover, the sharing that takes place among patients and their families provides a sense of support and strength through bonding. "I am not alone." "*We* are not alone." These messages—whether spoken or unspoken—do much to motivate patients to help each other, and therefore to help themselves.

Patient Participation in Informational/Supportive Programs

For cancer patients and their families to participate in informational and supportive programs gives them a sense of purpose.

Furthermore, it frequently allows the patient and family to speak together more openly about the disease and therefore to share their remaining days together more meaningfully, however numbered these may be. For many persons, association with other patients with cancer helps them to consolidate a sense of personal identity that is not morbidly entwined with their disease. Interpersonal bonds, both within and outside of the family, tend to be strengthened. Excessive denial of the disease and, in many cases, exaggerated denial of a tragically foreshortened life-span are also avoided by many patients who cope with their disease by sharing constructively with others.

In general, patients who participate in supportive and informational programs about cancer reach a state of acceptance more easily and find heightened pleasure in everyday tasks, recreation, and personal relationships. Of course, their energy is frequently limited because of the disease and/or its treatment. But what energy remains is more likely to be channeled into self-affirming activities. In our experience in the Mayo Cancer Rehabilitation Program, the outlook of patients tends to be less tinged with a sense of desperate urgency when they are helping one another; indeed, mutual support seems to foster heightened personality integration.

Role of the Medical Communications Specialist

As a medical communicator involved in the development of educational and supportive programs for patients with cancer and their families, I found that it was necessary to spend considerable time collaborating with cancer patients in the planning stages of any printed materials, audiovisual programs, or supportive programs if these programs were to prove worthwhile. A great lack, I found, lay in the failure of health care givers to appreciate fully the cognitive and affective needs of cancer patients and their families.[8] We on the health care team tended to second-guess what patients wanted to know, how they felt, and what kind of reassurance they wanted. Also, because some kinds of cancer are especially difficult for health care professionals to deal with, we often reacted with denial ourselves, thereby displacing onto patients our own anxieties and conflict avoidance. Only by the use of careful, thorough interviews and/or questionnaires, administered before the inception of any project designed for patient information or support, was it possible to proceed with confidence that the program would be successful. Thus, patient participation was required from the inception of a program to its completion.

This meant that every project went through an initial needs assessment phase. This usually consisted of interviewing between 10 and 30 patients (and, if possible, members of their families) with a particular form of cancer regarding their informational and supportive needs. Often, the initial interviews began with very general questions such as:

> Are there many things about your disease that you don't understand?
> What *do* you understand about your disease?
> What information would you like to have about your disease that you don't know now?
> Is there information that you would rather not know in detail?
> Would you find it helpful to have a booklet describing your disease and its treatment?
> Would you find it helpful to talk with other patients who have the same disease?

These are but a few examples. During the needs assessment phase, initial interviews (all audiotaped, with the permission of the patient) and/or questionnaires (a much less thorough means of obtaining information) were as open-ended as possible. This was necessary because specific questions usually generate specific answers—and if questions are too specific, much valuable information will be missed. Therefore, it was important during interviews that patients be given the widest possible latitude in describing their informational needs, their areas of anxiety, what they perceived their families' fears to be, how they viewed their disease, what kinds of information they thought would be helpful, what kinds of information would be anxiety-provoking, in what medium the information could be most effectively presented, and what kind of support they would find most helpful from health professionals, from other patients, and from family members.

Below is a description of a few of the approaches we used in the Cancer Rehabilitation Program of the Mayo Comprehensive Cancer Center during a period of funding from the National Cancer Institute between June 1974 and June 1977.[9] The approaches in each program were quite different, but all incorporated the precept that the patient must be an integral part of program planning and an essential determinant of what other patients' information and supportive needs really are. The development of a book on lung cancer for patients and their families is described below as a model project.

Patient Participation in Development of Lung Cancer Book

Origin of the Project. The idea for a book on lung cancer came from one of the co-authors of the book, D. T. Carr, who had specialized in the treatment of this disease for many years. The book was to be titled *Living with Lung Cancer: A Reference Book for People with Lung Cancer and Their Families.*[10] This physician had received repeated requests over the years from his patients for reading materials about lung cancer, but nothing appropriate was available in public libraries or bookstores. Patients had access only to lengthy, highly technical descriptions that appeared in medical textbooks, leaving them more confused than ever; they even resorted to medical dictionaries.[11] A scattering of popular books about cancer was available, but these were far too general for most patients.

Needs Assessment Phase. My work began with the needs assessment phase of the book. This meant conducting tape-recorded interviews of lung cancer patients and their spouses to determine what these individuals wanted to know about lung cancer, and especially what they thought should be included in the book. The transcripts of these interviews formed the basis for the initial draft of the book manuscript. The next step consisted of lengthy tape-recorded interviews of the various health professionals involved in the care of patients with lung cancer. These individuals provided the bulk of technical information for the book. Medical textbooks were consulted, as well.

Development of the Manuscript. When I had compiled the information from all of these sources and had written the first rough draft of *Living with Lung Cancer*, the manuscript was submitted for review to 20 physicians (medical oncologists) who were experts in the treatment of cancer. They made certain that the medical content was correct before the manuscript was re-reviewed by lung cancer patients and their spouses.

Over 20 patients with lung cancer and members of their families acted as the final arbiters of the content and tone of the book. They reviewed the manuscript in detail. Each filled out a questionnaire about the information in the book, addressing the material paragraph by paragraph. They also penciled suggested revisions directly on the manuscript pages. When this task was completed, I interviewed them at length about their responses to the manuscript. We later transcribed these tape-recorded sessions, which provided us with the information necessary for final revision of the book. My interviews with these patients and their families revealed that countless questions about lung cancer were never asked in the doctor's office. Patients had many reasons for not asking questions. "The doctor is so busy." "It seemed like a dumb question to ask." "I was embarrassed to bring that up." "I always seemed to forget my questions until the doctor left the office." There were a myriad of other reasons why patients found it difficult to ask questions in the doctor's office. During our interviews, however, they stated that they badly needed background information to help them cope with their lung cancer, its treatment, and, particularly, their nameless fears about the future.

Patient Evaluation of Manuscript. When patients with lung cancer and their families reviewed the last draft of the book, we were relieved to find that they were both critical and thorough— not only in their suggestions regarding the content, but in their recommendations about the "tone" of the text. In effect, they told us how to talk on paper most comfortably and effectively to other cancer patients. Their honesty was partly due to our repeated assurances that I, as a medical communications specialist, was not a participant in their health care. Moreover, I had no influence upon the care given to them by physicians, nurses, and other health professionals. Their anonymity in their communications with me was also assured. Therefore, they had license to be honest without fear of consequences.

As a medical communications specialist, I feel convinced from my experience in clinical settings that patients withhold many questions from physicians because of their dependency relationship and because of fears of abandonment. They frequently feel that they must "please" the physician and other health care givers, lest they receive suboptimal care or, worse yet, are subtly rejected because of the stress their disease (cancer) places both on them and on the health professionals around them.

Yet, most patients and their families will communicate their needs openly with a third person (e.g., a medical communications specialist) not directly involved in their medical care. Under these conditions, patients usually divulge considerable information about their psychological and learning needs.

The book *Living with Lung Cancer* was essentially edited from cover to cover *by* patients *for* patients. They recognized how desperately they had wanted information about their disease when they were going through the stage of shock after diagnosis and through the stresses of therapy. As a result, they wanted to help other patients who followed them to be better informed, and therefore better equipped to deal with their disease. Consequently, the patients who participated in the writing of *Living with Lung Cancer* gave long hours of their time to the development of the book. By their words and by their actions, these individuals reinforced our belief that patients and their families want and need to share information in order to cope with the physical and psychological problems that accompany lung cancer and its treatment. They recognized that knowledge is a weapon against cancer, and they wanted to pass this weapon on to other patients.

Other Informational and Counseling Projects

The participation of patients and their families proved equally effective in a number of other patient information and counseling programs in the Mayo Cancer Rehabilitation Program. These programs, too, were based on the premise that any patient information counseling program will fail unless it is based on the needs of the patient as they are perceived by the patient, as well as by the involved health professionals. As in the model project described above, patients' needs were assessed by questioning them in a way that avoided their confronting the health care professionals upon whom they depended for care.

Below is described a sampling of rehabilitation programs conducted as part of the Mayo Comprehensive Cancer Center's Rehabilitation Program.

Enterostomal Rehabilitation Program. In the Enterostomal Program, patients were active in a number of projects. Among the more important of these was a book describing a new surgical procedure, the continent ileostomy. [12,13] Because so little was known about the long-term sequelae of this procedure, it was necessary to have the input of patients. Health professionals simply did not have the data; patients did. Consequently, before the book was written, 12 patients who had undergone the continent ileostomy responded to a lengthy needs assessment questionnaire concerning all aspects of their adjustment—both physical and psychological. Their ideas shaped the content of the first draft of the book. Upon completion of this draft, approximately 40 additional patients reviewed the manuscript in detail, suggesting changes and additions and completing a long, detailed survey form. As my co-author and I stated in the foreword of the book:

> This booklet has many authors. Two people put the words on paper, but all of the ideas on the pages that follow came from a host of contributors: surgeons, internists, enterostomal therapists—and most important of all, patients themselves. . . . All of the patients who participated in this project were tough honest editors and critics. They wanted to speak through us to you, the reader. So we listened, we rewrote, and we polished the material until it reflected the real, day-to-day experiences of the person with an ileal pouch. [12]

Patients who had undergone other types of ostomy surgery participated in the planning of programs, as well. For example, they critiqued films produced by various organizations for colostomy patients. Films receiving highly favorable reviews were then shown on closed-circuit television at scheduled times to hospitalized patients who had just undergone this surgery. Another project was patient evaluation of an annual conference entitled "Ostomy Update." Participants in the conference consisted of ostomates, their spouses, nurses, enterostomal therapists, physicians, and other health professionals. At the conclusion of the conference, evaluations were conducted of all participants, and the resulting data determined the format for the program the following year. In this way, patients had an important voice in the educational opportunities that would be made available to other patients in the future.

Cancer Amputee Rehabilitation Program. A Cancer Amputee Program was another important component of the Cancer Rehabilitation Program. One of the outcomes of this program, based on collaboration among patients, health professionals, and medical communications specialists, was a film entitled *The Road to Recovery*. The content of this film was initially determined by numerous audiotaped interviews with cancer amputees—generally young people with osteogenic sarcoma—and their parents. It became evident from the interviews that patients wanted to see other cancer amputees who had recovered successfully and had resumed active normal lives. Consequently, we selected as the "star" of our film a 16-year-old girl, a lower-extremity cancer amputee, who had undergone amputation one year previously at a Mayo-affiliated hospital. Her mother also appeared in the film. The film depicted the diagnostic stage, preoperative preparation, immediate postoperative course, and the lengthy rehabilitation process that follows amputation of a lower limb. Scenes of the surgery itself were eliminated, because patients wished not to see this; it was too frightening and traumatic. At the conclusion of the film, scenes of several cancer amputees of various ages were shown as they engaged in various sports. This offered added reassurance to the amputee viewers that males and females of all ages were capable of regaining adequate function—in many cases nearly normal function.

Another project in the Cancer Amputee Program was an "Amputee Visitor Program." This program, fashioned after the American Cancer Society's "Reach to Recovery" program, consisted of recovered cancer amputee volunteers who came to the hospital to visit other cancer patients upon whom amputation had just been performed. It was our experience that, approximately two to seven days after surgery, cancer amputees were particularly subject to feelings of depression and despondency regarding their future. No reassurance from the medical staff could convince them that they would be able to walk normally again and resume their accustomed activities. A pilot study of our "Amputee Visitor Program" established that visits by recovered amputees had a dramatic positive effect on the morale of patients who had just undergone operation. The amputee visitors served not only as important role models for the patient, but also were able to give patients information about and perspective on the long and complex rehabilitation process.

Conclusion

Patients with cancer are greatly helped in their adjustment to their disease, and even to their impending death, by being allowed to help other patients. They participate effectively in the development of printed materials, audiovisual programs, counseling programs, and psychological support programs. The cancer patients who are the recipients of such programs are obviously helped, as well, because they have the benefit of the input, sensitivity, and knowledge of other cancer patients who have gone through the same experience and who understand best their informational and supportive needs.

References

1. Lazes, P. M. Health education project guides outpatients to active self-care. *Hospitals, J.A.H.A.* 51:81–86, 1977.
2. Wang, V. L., Reiter, H., Lentz, G. A., Jr., and Whaples, G. C. An approach to consumer-patient activation in health maintenance. *Public Health Reports* 90: 449–454, 1975.
3. Janik, N. The shortest distance between treatment and survival: Reach to recovery. *Proceedings of The American Cancer Society Second National Conference on Human Values & Cancer*, Chicago, 1977, pp. 180–182.
4. *1977 Cancer Facts & Figures*. New York: American Cancer Society, 1976, pp. 24–25.
5. Yahle, M. E. An ostomy information clinic. *Nurs. Clin. North Am.* 11:457–467, 1975.
6. Kelly, O. E. Make Today Count. In: *National Cancer Institute Response Book*, Bethesda, National Cancer Institute, 1978, paragraph 9.12.
7. Monaco, M. *The Candlelighters: Parents Dedicated to the Conquest of Cancer*. Washington D.C.: Candlelighters, 1972.
8. Levin, L. S. Patient education and self-care: How do they differ? *Nurs. Outlook* 26:170–175, 1978.
9. Cox, B. G. The fine art of educating the patient. *Med. Opinion* 4:31–35, 1975.
10. Cox, B. G., Carr, D. T., and Lee, R. E. *Living with Lung Cancer: A Reference Book for People with Lung Cancer and Their Families*. Rochester, Minn.: Mayo Foundation, 1977.

11. Roth, B. G. Health information for patients: The hospital library's role. *Bull. Med. Libr. Assoc.*66:14–17, 1978.

12. Cox, B. G., and Wentworth, A. A. *The Ileal Pouch Procedure: A New Outlook for the Person with an Ileostomy.* Rochester, Minn.: Mayo Foundation, 1975.

13. Cox, B. G., and Wentworth, A. A. An evaluation model for the development of patient education literature. *Biosciences Communications*2:333–341, 1976.

8

Anticipatory Grief, Stress, and the Surrogate Griever

Robert Fulton, Ph.D.

There is nothing like a little stress to enhance our well-being. Stress can serve as a force for growth, or if nothing else it can clear the air. Permit me to respond to the somewhat contending points of view expressed by Dr. Mount and Dr. Luthe.

I believe we should bear in mind that the prospect of death can be very stressful, painful, and difficult not only for the very young but for the old also. We must not forget that we can become so immersed in what we do, and so caught up in what we believe, that eventually we reach a point of assuming that what we do is right and that what is right is what we do! I do not think we should forget that there are other perceptions and definitions of reality besides our own.

In this regard, I believe we can gain valuable insights by historical and cross-cultural analysis of the ways in which people throughout the world deal with death. Among certain South-West Indians, for example, there is total avoidance of the dead. On the other hand, in more than a dozen societies scattered around the

Robert Fulton • Professor of Sociology and Director, Center for Death Education and Research, University of Minnesota, Minneapolis, Minnesota 55455.

world, the dead are ceremoniously eaten by the survivors. I have absolutely no knowledge of what the long-term consequences of eating a corpse are for the survivors. I do know, however, that it is important for us to recognize that the spectrum of human behavior, with regard to the dead, ranges from abhorence of the corpse and abandonment of the body to the eating of it. When we deliberate about death, we cannot afford to disregard the cultural variations that can and do exist.

With this caveat in mind, I would like to share certain ideas about stress as it relates to the care of the dying patient. To do this, however, I first wish to say something about our contemporary experiences with—and our attitudes toward—death.

The categories of death are expanding in our society. The conception of death—or more correctly the conception of life—has changed. That is, in contrast to the recent past, the conception of life has contracted while death has extended its parameters over life. Who is considered alive and who is considered dead is not as clear-cut as it once was. Viability has been foreshortened.

Formerly life began with conception. With the Supreme Court's ruling that a fetus is not "alive" until after the 21st week of gestation, "life" has had to pull at its belt. Our societal attitudes toward death, it would appear, are beginning to parallel the views of life and death found among some non-Western societies, in which not only are the dead dead, but the elderly and the very ill are dead also, while the unborn are not considered to be of this world.

Moreover, the definition of death itself has changed from just a decade ago. Until quite recently, death was something you could put your finger on, so to speak. You could check a patient's eye for a light reaction, feel his pulse, test for respiration, or prick his skin. Failing a response, you could reasonably conclude that he was dead. Today, however, there are organ transplant programs and other medical procedures that frequently make it necessary to run an EEG to be certain that a patient is "brain dead."

The increased complexity of death is also reflected in the new issues and dilemmas surrounding grief and bereavement. One of the most fruitful approaches to our understanding of human response to loss was initiated by Lindemann at Massachusetts General Hospital in the 1940's. His studies, simple as they were, were profound in their implications and illuminating in terms of our systematic understanding of the nature of grief. It was he, in fact, who first coined the expression "anticipatory grief." Because of him, we can not only talk about normal grief in a new light but also about pathologic grief, chronic grief, anticipatory grief, and surrogate grief.

The domain of bereavement is well worth exploring— particularly the question of whether grief is natural to man, or whether it is a consequence of cultural conditioning. The question was raised over 30 years ago by Spiro, an anthropologist who worked among the Ifaluk. He observed that while family members displayed considerable pain and discomfort when a family member died, they were able to smile and laugh and generally act as if they had suffered no loss once the funeral was over. It was as if their grief had disappeared by magic.

Spiro's work flies in the face of what common sense would tell us about grief, and it challenges as well those studies of both humans and animals that weigh in favor of a genetically determined grief response. At best, we can only say at this time that the issue of nature versus nurture with regard to the grief reaction remains unresolved. What we do know, however, is that when it comes to an immediate response to separation by death, people tend to react differently.

Observed variations in the response to separation by death permit us to make a distinction between what can be termed a "high-grief" death and a "low-grief" death. If the expression "low-grief" can be allowed to describe the reaction to the death of many elderly persons today, "high-grief" describes the impact of a death—brought about suddenly or unexpectedly—of a person on whom others depend heavily for their social and psychological well-being. Such a death usually precipitates a series of intense emotional and physical reactions that we recognize as the "normal grief" syndrome.

Experience with death, grief, and bereavement in modern urban societies has changed significantly over the past decades. At the turn of the century, for example, over half of all deaths in the United States were those of children under 15 years of age. Today, death is increasingly an experience of the aged. If I were to show you a graph of the present mortality of American society, it would be much like a J-curve. Under one year of age, there is an appreciable rate of mortality, but this flattens out until nearly the fifth decade of life, when a sharp rise begins. Separation and loss experiences follow a similar pattern. We should note that the greatest number of those who die in our society today are the elderly. For those of us in the middle years, we are, in a sense, death-insulated. As for the young people of our society, their chances are only 5 per 100 that they will have any direct immediate experience with death within their nuclear families before they attain their 21st year.

In the majority of cases, it is the elderly who die; moreover, they die from diseases quite dissimilar from those which once killed children. The elderly die from heart disease, stroke, cancer, and other degenerative diseases associated with the aging process. In this sense, death today is different from any death that has ever previously been experienced by society. Men and women die under the care of highly skilled medical functionaries in segregated hospital communities. And they die for reasons that, by and large, were—statistically speaking—unknown two or three generations ago. At the turn of the century, for instance, only 4% of the population was over 65 years of age; they represented 17% of all deaths. Today, the elderly represent 11% of the population but contribute over 70% of the deaths. In the majority of cases, moreover, they die in a hospital or in a setting other than their own homes.

It is important to note, also, that the contemporary setting within which the majority of people die has brought about profound changes in the level of emotional reaction to loss, as well as a change in those who share the loss. Research has shown that, frequently, professional caregivers experience grief at the loss of a patient and in many other ways react like bereaved survivors themselves. As the traditional kinship network falters or as family members disengage from their relationship with the dying patient, the attending nurse and other care givers frequently find themselves participating in the social and emotional support of patients under their care. Such involvement—albeit at times inadvertent—

brings with it a new responsibility, as it involves new emotional risks. In fact, as Mary Vachon has informed us, she and her colleagues at the Clark Institute in Toronto have found that the stress level of critical care nurses is often as high as the stress levels of the patients for whom they care.

That this could occur is made possible not only by the circumstances of modern life that have given rise to a whole new health industry for the care of the elderly, but occurs also because of a phenomenon called "anticipatory grief." This term refers to the fact that the patient's death is anticipated prior to its actual occurrence and that there is an accommodation that goes on among the survivors and health-care personnel in expectation of what is to happen. Studies have shown that in some instances—where it was observed that family members were withdrawing physically and emotionally from a patient—health care personnel became caught up in the patient's life. New emotional bonds were established, with the result that the health care team members found themselves grieved persons when the patient died. Thus, the phenomenon of anticipatory grief helps turn professional caregivers into grievers, or what I have termed "surrogate grievers."

With what result? I believe the phenomenon gives rise to the potential for role discrepancy and role reversal on the part of the caregiver and the survivor. The caregiver grieves but is not bereaved, while the bereft survivor may be beyond experiencing his or her grief. Thus, the role of the surrogate griever not only has the capacity for complicating the dying process, but it has the potential also for casting into a bad light the muted responses or misunderstood reactions of the immediate survivor. For example, I remember an incident at Wayne State University some years ago when a group of physicians, nurses, and paramedical personnel met to discuss this issue. A nurse jumped up and said with great emotion "If family survivors can't behave the way they should following a death, they should stay away from the hospital and from the funeral!" To repeat: it can happen that by the time the death of the patient occurs, the staff will experience the loss of the patient more deeply than expected, while a confused mother—not understanding her lack of affect or her inability to cry or express her grief—will attempt to act out the role of hostess! Thus, it happens that her behavior is misinterpreted by the staff, and she is perceived as being heartless.

A case in point is the physician's wife who lost her husband to cancer of the abdomen. He had originally experimented on himself at a medical school, ingesting radioactive fats as part of his work toward a Ph.D. thesis on carcinogenic substances. Two-and-a-half years later, as he was about to graduate, he became ill, and his cancer was subsequently diagnosed. A university medical team decided to film his dying for educational purposes, recording the events that occurred between him and his wife, as well as videotaping a series of interviews with a psychiatrist colleague.

Over the four- to five-month period that the interviews were conducted, the wife's appearance changed dramatically. Initially, she wore her long hair severely pulled back, dark horn-rimmed glasses, long skirts, and "sensible" shoes. By the end of the interviews she had become "Vogue-like" in appearance—just the opposite of the image she had first presented the viewer. Neither she nor the psychiatrist acknowledged this change, nor were they conscious of talking about her husband in the *past tense* (even though at the time he was very much alive). They never realized the mental shift that had occurred to them both. I would argue that the phenomenon of anticipatory grief played a very important part in the change in the wife's physical appearance, as well as in her emotional transformation. One is left to imagine how she thought of herself or what others who knew them both thought of her appearance or behavior at the time of her husband's death.

Increasingly, studies have investigated the role of the caregiver in relationship to dying patients. Let me mention one that deals not with the dying of an elderly patient, but rather with the death of children from leukemia. The Natterson–Knudson study was conducted 15 years ago at City of Hope, Duarte, California. In their study, a scenario that was repeated in different cases went something as follows:

A mother would bring a child into the hospital after having sought out one physician after another to reassure her that the child did *not* have leukemia. Finally, on recognizing that the child *had* to be hospitalized, the mother would come into the hospital clutching the child. She would insist on remaining with the child. She would become consumed by the child's illness. She would leave her husband—and other children if there were any—in favor of the sick child. Over a period of months, however, as the child and mother settled into the hospital routine, she would begin to yield. Slowly she would remove herself from the child and the hospital and return to her family. She would visit her child less frequently; and often when she did return to the hospital, she would come with an article from a medical journal or an account of a new treatment or procedure and discuss the contents with the child's physician. Her preoccupation with her child's illness became a preoccupation with leukemia wherever it appeared throughout the world. She began to transcend or sublimate her experience. Finally—in terms of her involvement, emotional expressions of affection, or time spent with the child—there was an observable decline. There were fewer tears shed, but more abstract discussions on the nature of the disease. Contact with other children in the ward was initiated. New areas of interest opened up for her. Ultimately, when she lost all hope, she questioned the value of continuing the treatments. Surprising for all, it was now the attending physician who argued for the treatment to be continued or new procedures initiated! A reversal in roles had taken place. Suddenly, the physician had taken on the role of the mother—as she had first appeared to him—while the mother had assumed the role of the physician.

Anticipatory grief may be either a personal or collective response to stress. Given the peculiarities of illnesses among the elderly, like cancer—especially with its capacity for prolonging dying—anticipatory grief introduces a whole new dimension of stress for family members and caregivers alike. For family members who have to deal with the separation and loss of their loved one, the stressful event can be muted and possibly sublimated. On the other hand, professional care givers may find an *increase* in the amount of stress they must endure.

In summary, it is important to recognize that a new phenomenon is among us. It results from human beings dying in segregated institutions staffed by specialized care givers. Such a situation has the potential to reverse the role between surviving family members and health care personnel. This reversal has major implications for the level of stress that may be experienced by all concerned.

9

Bereavement: Including Some Iatrogenic Aspects of Grief

Terence E. Lear, F.R.C.P.I., D.P.M., F.R.C.Psych.

Separation

The sorrow of parting, unless brief, is not at all sweet, in my experience. I can reflect that while a parting is not as final as a death, it may yet prepare me for the grief associated with death. An understanding of the grief associated with separation should be a topic included in medical education, because the implications of grief for the medical profession are widespread. The painstaking work of John Bowlby (1953) and Colin Murray Parkes (1972) made clear that the loss of separation provokes similar symptoms, whether the loss is temporary—as when a mother leaves her child in the hospital—or permanent, as when a person suffers a bereavement. Other losses, too, cause suffering similar to that of bereavement, although close observations have shown some differences in detail. In disregarding these differences, I meet objections of over-inclusiveness with the plea that this does at least provide an opportunity to review some of our medical practices.

Terence E. Lear • Physician and Consultant Psychiatrist, St. Crispin Hospital, Northampton, England NN2 6JF.

Any baby can expect feeding and stimulation from his mother. Good-enough mothering promotes tolerance of brief absences of the mother, but prolonged separation is associated with certain changes in the child, which were described graphically by Bowlby and portrayed in a series of moving films made by the Robertsons (1967–1976).

Just as a child can use almost any materials in play to represent what is inside him, so what happens externally must somehow be represented inside. Thus, one could talk about a mother external to the child or the child's inner representation of mother. When I use the term *psychosocial experience*, I mean to include both sorts of experience. The psychosocial experience of a child separated from his mother can be described as follows:

The child searches high and low for his mother. He is resentful that she is not there. There are rest periods but the search continues in vain until at last he gives up. Then he feels hopeless, defeated, and alone. Later he picks himself up and gets to know others around him. Those others may get a hint that he is not quite all there. The three stages observed in the child on which this is based are anger, apathy, and detachment. They are accompanied by somatic and psychological symptoms. If the child becomes reunited with his mother, some aspects of these stages become manifest again, and for some time the child does not easily let his mother out of view or reach.

Grief

In the introduction to his book *Bereavement (Studies of Grief in Adult Life)* (1972), Colin Murray Parkes writes, "Grief, like any other aspect of human behavior, is capable of description and study and, when studied, it turns out to be as fascinating as any other psychological phenomenon." That is certainly how his book reads. He lists the following seven aspects of reaction to bereavement:

- Realization, in which the bereaved moves from denial or avoidance of recognition of the loss to acceptance of it.

- An alarm reaction: anxiety, restlessness, and the physiological concomitants of fear.
- The urge to search for, and to find, the lost person in some way.
- Anger and guilt, including outbursts directed against those who press the bereaved person toward premature acceptance of his loss.
- Feeling of internal loss or of mutilation of self.
- Identification phenomena: the adoption of traits, mannerisms, or symptoms of the lost person, with or without a sense of his presence within the self.
- Pathological variants of grief, in which the reaction may be excessive and prolonged or inhibited and inclined to emerge in distorted form.

To these we can add "the gaining of a new identity," meaning that through resignation the bereaved accepts life without the lost one, thus becoming in effect a different person.

All the stages of separation are contained in this listing.

Symptomatology

The symptomatology of grief is interesting because its genesis is twofold. Those symptoms which can be connected with somatic disorders are easy for doctors to conceptualize. The common somatic effects produced by stress are mediated by the autonomic system, which supplies smooth muscle and endocrine glands. These somatic effects in turn provoke further psychological distress, which can then lead to still further somatic effects, creating a vicious cycle. The list of these effects is very long: trembling, loss of appetite and weight, sweating, fatigue, insomnia, palpitations, over-breathing, dry mouth, blurred vision, headaches, dizziness, faints, chest pains, aches, menorrhagia, digestive upsets, vomiting, rheumatism, asthma, skin rashes, nightmares, restlessness, depression, poor memory and concentration, difficulty with decisions, irritability, tension, panic feelings, fears of heavy drinking, nocturnal orgasms, sense of unreality, and suicidal ideas of low intensity. During bereavement, there is some proneness to organic disease such as infections, coronary thrombosis, cervical and blood cancers, and arthritis. Symptoms then develop from the organ dysfunctions brought about by these disorders.

The other category of symptoms which the bereaved person may develop consists of those which bear a striking similarity to the symptoms of the one who died. These are psychologically created by the bereaved himself. Home (1966) talks of Freud's discovery that physical symptoms can have meaning in the context of the personal life of the patient, and that these symptoms are therefore personal creations rather than being the effects of causes.

Temporary respite from the pain of loss may be won by the bereaved creating and retaining (inside himself) all or part of the lost person and specifically that person's suffering. Sometimes the dead person is seen or heard, so intense is the synthesis of past and present perceptions.

Dying

The dying person, too, slowly loses all that life means to him and suffers his own grief. It is not surprising, then, to find similar reactions in experiences of dying. These experiences are described by Elizabeth Kübler-Ross in her book *On Death and Dying* (1970). She had the brilliant idea of meeting with patients who were dying in a General Hospital, together with medical students, the hospital chaplain, and sometimes nurses, and asking their assistance in understanding a dying person's needs. The mutual help of dying person and relatives, and dying person and professional helpers, became apparent. Many (but not all) of the dying were relieved to have the opportunity to *talk* about dying. This was Hinton's experience (1967) too when he visited people dying in the hospital. It is possible to talk about dying without depriving all hope of recovery from the dying person. Their work suggests that, in some cases, doctors are more reluctant to offer the patients the opportunity to talk than the patients are to initiate a discussion. This results in a lack of encouragement for the dying person and relatives to do grief work together. The reluctance of the doctor is due to his uncertainties of his own feelings. In such circumstances, one possibility is to share the experience by talking with at least one other professional colleague, or even visiting jointly. Thinking of the dying person as the best ally of the grieving relatives is a useful view. This suggests one reason why relatives are so disadvantaged in the event of *sudden death*. Getting accustomed to the idea, and recognizing death only with great difficulty when a person dies suddenly, shows through in the ancient practice of burying persons who commit suicide near a crossroads with a stake through the heart. It is as if passersby must bear witness that the body is truly dead and will not rise to haunt them. The idea of the Cross affording protection may be in this as well, perhaps? Relatives who have to cope with sudden deaths often are shocked and numbed at first and their grief is that more serious and in need of help. This is at a time when the doctor may be taken by surprise too. It is a strange paradox that the doctor's resources may be reduced when his patient needs them most. Perhaps clergymen and social workers might be more aware of the need to rally around when somone dies suddenly. This may be so with unexpected deaths in a hospital ward.

Developmental and unusual events influence everyone in the family and constitute a crisis of change involving a sort of bereavement process. The examples following clarify this statement.

Stillbirth

Bourne (1968), using a questionnaire method, investigated 100 cases of stillbirth compared with 100 live births from the observations of family doctors. While the psychological effects on the mother and family were interesting, it was even more striking and statistically significant that the doctors did not seem to know, notice, or remember anything about the patient who had the stillbirth. Bourne describes stillbirth as a *nonevent*, since it is not an illness which can be accepted or treated, and the bereaved have no familiar human being to mourn. A stillbirth is relatively rare, public knowledge, and occurs after pregnancy and preparation have been obvious and in progress for months. By contrast, an abortion follows a short gestation; the fetus is so tiny that without a good look it is unrecognizable as a human; and the event is private and commonplace.

Bourne suggests that doctors may be at a loss confronting a patient withdrawing into shame and anger who may have little inclination to talk. He warns against urging another pregnancy as therapy. A new pregnancy is likely to complicate the grief work for the failed pregnancy, and the patient may be unable to cope with such a complexity of events, so that severe symptoms and even a psychotic breakdown occurs. He counsels doctors to learn how to put the optimum distance between themselves and patients, and he advocates more reporting of follow-up observations to stillbirth in the medical literature.

Lewis (1976) responded to Bourne by relating some of his own experiences with stillbirths in the hospital. Taking up Bourne's challenge, he submitted his own recommendations about the management of these cases. He noted, by way of analogy, that the mourning of someone missing and presumed killed was difficult during and after the World Wars, and that this problem was ameliorated by the Tomb to the Unknown Warrior. He continues: "There is an added sense of unreality with stillbirths as there are no experiences with the baby to remember. Looking at and holding the dead baby, giving the baby a name, arranging the certification, attending the funeral, and knowing its grave help to make stillbirths a reality to the family. With these activities memories are created which aid the recovery processes of mourning."

He observes that following a stillbirth, there is a conspiracy of silence between doctor and patient which, although well-meaning on both sides, tends to confirm the mother's shame and guilt based on her fantasies that the baby's death was a consequence of her own thoughts or deeds. By concealing her distress, she protects the doctor, evades facing up to her loss, and deprives herself of the talk with him and others which can assist her during mourning. He recommends that hospital staffs should discourage a woman from this sort of isolation by expressing their own sadness about her stillbirth to the patient.

Pregnancy and Childbirth

In the same paper, Lewis offers another gem: the concept of "the baby inside." Caplan (1961) described in great detail the experiences of women adjusting from pregnancy to motherhood, and the complexities of the physiological, psychological, and social changes for them in relating to a new baby. The attention the prospective mother receives during pregnancy is bound to be missed after childbirth occurs. These are rather abstract notions, however, and less pertinent to our discussion than the loss of the baby inside—and the void this creates—after birth. I know that many mothers remain puzzled years afterwards as to why their joy with a new baby was mingled with sadness. Of course, when a stillbirth takes place, there is a double loss—inside *and* outside— and hence double grief.

That there is grief associated with live births may come as a surprise to some doctors who, nevertheless, should have no difficulty in recognizing it in their clinical observations. Recognition of grief should help them to comfort the bereaved mother after confinement. I wonder if the husband's participation at confinement can help? They, too, may suffer grief as well (presumably, Couvade's syndrome is an intensification of the normal father experience.)

Menopause

The "change of life" is accompanied by loss of ovulation and menstruation with associated hormonal changes. This is a bald physiological principle, contrasting with the complexity of presenting clinical experience. When the physical changes are slow and indistinct, psychological aspects may be out of phase, particularly when family experience is so varied. Thus, a woman at this time of life may feel very differently about such changes if she still has young children than if her children are teenagers.

The changes may be anticipated by years, and a sense of impending loss can be puzzling and terrifying. For instance, a woman with a much older partner may feel she draws nearer her husband's age as he gets older. Again as her husband gets older, he comes to resemble her father more and more. There may be an interplay of feelings about loss and psychosexual experience. With the menopause, memories of her menarche are stirred, particularly if there is a daughter at puberty or adolescence in the family.

Listening to a woman talking lyrically about pregnancy, childbirth, and baby craft, I have asked, "Are you thinking of starting another baby?" And she retorts with, "Our family is complete, that would be absurd." In other words, *she* does the reality testing. In other cases, I may be asked, Do you think that we should start another baby?" In which case, *I* do the reality testing by asking her to look at the consequences. It is tempting for a woman to embark on an unwanted pregnancy, sometimes at the doctor's suggestion. When there is menorrhagia, the idea that an operation would remove the trouble can be appealing. A troublesome symptom may be removed by hysterectomy, but this would be an organ loss added to other losses.

On the other hand, I remember as a student a gynecologist who described to his patients a Manchester repair: "You are going to have a vagina like a young woman of 17." In this way he defined the limit of loss; the underlying message was that while the vagina might no longer be the instrument for delivering a baby, it would still be an effectual organ for pleasure.

Marriage

Marital work involves each partner working through the grief associated with the loss of significant people in his or her past. Perhaps the resolution may be inconclusive but the effort is toward *some* resolution. The pain of loss can be mitigated by visualizing in the partner a parent or other important person from the past. Each partner may use these means to remain comforted, and tacitly they agree not to notice how they are relating. The cost of the arrangement is likely to be hesitancy at lovemaking and parenthood, since one or the other partner may either identify with, or feel rivalry toward, a child in the family. Eventually, new ways of relating involve a new identity and perhaps, role, for each partner. Just as a doctor would not expect his patient's grief to go away quickly, so a couple who are trying to understand their marriage will want to take time over it. To know that the doctor is aware of their distress and is available for consultation may be enough. Others may prefer to have regular sessions individually or jointly with an experienced counselor.

With anticipated or actual separation, there is the loss of the actual partner, but the opportunity is lost, too, of projecting on to the partner the needed people from inner to outer experience. There may be a loss of status and sometimes concomitant loss of parenthood and home, together with a challenge of a new identity and role to assume. It is not surprising that frequently this distress is circumvented by precipitate involvement with another partner reminiscent of the first.

The doctor would do his patient no service by advising him to find another partner—or to marry one he has found already, too soon—just to assuage his grief.

Breaks in the Doctor/Patient Relationship

"Love at first sight" is an expression which connotes two people getting involved and becoming dependent upon each other almost instantaneously. A patient undergoing psychotherapy can also become childlike in session, and his therapist becomes immensely important to his life. Part of the treatment is to discuss this dependency and to make allowances for separations at holidays and at the end of treatment. Thus, by ordered preparation for separation, personal growth occurs. The provision of suitable conditions is the responsibility of the doctor or social worker. Otherwise the patient's feelings of abandonment may be intolerable.

Patients in distress quickly become involved with a doctor, social worker, or nurse. If the patient does not understand the working arrangements under which he may sometimes be served by different attendants than the one to whom he has become attached—there may be a terrible sense of loss added to his other troubles. There are occasions when nurses are moved from one ward to another, one doctor covers for another, or a social worker goes off call after the weekend; at these times, a patient can feel stranded. Sometimes, if the patient is informed at the beginning, he himself can limit his involvement in a single interview. At other times, the best work may lie in clarifying who may be available to see the experience through with the patient. The hospital atmosphere does influence patients towards regression so that there may be some pressure from the patient to tell the hospital doctor personal troubles. I suppose the art lies in listening to a bit and then spending some of the time contacting the patient's general practitioner, rather than ignoring personal communications and concentrating solely on the physical condition, on the one hand, or getting unrealistically entangled on the other.

Sometimes a patient goes to another doctor when her own is away and she requires medical consultation. Or she is referred to a different psychiatrist when the psychiatrist she usually sees goes on a holiday. Unless the separation is understood as truly upsetting, the doctor covering may not make a fuss of her for a short time, to tide over, but makes alternative arrangements which cause a good treatment opportunity to be lost to her. Many doctors seem surprised when I suggest that a group member is going to get upset during a holiday break in group treatment. They may concur with the patient at these times that the treatment is not doing any good and change it. This is more prone to occur early in the group treatment because later on the patient understands more the nature of these experiences.

The Inquest

Parkes (1972) found that among various bereaved patients undergoing psychiatric treatment, about one-quarter showed considerable animosity toward the doctor or clergyman. Even among widows who experience usual grief reactions, most had periods of bitterness and irritability in which they tended to blame others.

A doctor, nurse, or social worker who has been involved with a patient has his or her own burden of grief. They, too, may question their treatment or care—"could I have done more?" This makes them particularly vulnerable to criticism; the remonstrations of relatives or a coroner's inquest can loom as a very threatening experience. In fact, these are an occasion for reality testing; and nearly always, doctors and relatives alike come to see that responsible care for the deceased was forthcoming from relatives and doctors. The skill of the coroner lies in questioning in such a way that the cause of death is clarified and that no unwarranted blame attaches to anyone for this. It is not easy for doctors to acknowledge publicly that their skills have limits when their hopes may have been otherwise. The concealment of these limits would give a false impression of negligence. The overscrupulous coroner who does not see the relationship between the grief and criticism of relatives, and takes the latter at face value, may find flaws in a doctor's practice. Doctors are human after all. Nonetheless, public accountability is important and serious negligence does occur. I believe, however, that such negligence is rather rare compared with the frequent accusations of negligence that are made after a death. At inquests, and more generally, the doctor can pause and consider that—uncomfortable as accusations are—they can be countered with a dispassionate statement of facts, and moreover that this reflects an unpleasant phase of mourning which will pass. It may be a partner in the practice or a district nurse who hears the criticisms of the bereaved person about the doctor who attended the deceased. It is very hard sometimes not to retaliate when attacked, but one of the best therapeutic maxims is "survive the attacks." The attacks may be acknowledged as such but what counts and is most therapeutic is the doctor's survival, namely that he is still there and available. Retaliation makes the doctor relatively unavailable, thereby increasing the bereaved person's loss. The benefit of sharing experiences with partners or other professional colleagues is great at these times. "Ungrateful so-and-so's," coming from a colleague, can be balm.

Loss of Home

Often the environment of an old person has been reduced to the home in which he lives with a spouse, a family member, or alone. The familiar sights, sounds, touch and smells of home and belongings seem all-important. Home is mother. Leaving home to live elsewhere must be a terrible loss for such an old person. When admitted to a hospital ward or nursing home, the old person becomes restless, wanders, shows truculence or apathy, which is regarded as a confusional state rather than grief. If the true nature of the patient's disaffection is not understood by the staff, they feel unable to cope with the situation, and may resort to the administration of drugs which slow the patient's awareness of the new surroundings, and also the contact with people who may help her back to the familiar experience which remains to her. General practitioners and social workers have often argued that the confusion was present before the person left home. This may be because of *anticipatory grief*—offers of stays elsewhere or knowledge of an elderly neighbor or relative losing a home can be a catalyst for this. Physical causes which disturb a person's awareness require detection, and perceptual loss itself must arouse grief. Besides physical causes, however, seeking recent and anticipated losses can be very rewarding in understanding an old person's confusion.

To send an old person away from home is so serious that the question of when and how such arrangements should occur needs care, particularly if the person is already bereaved. Often at weekends when on call, I have calls from general practitioners or social workers with the comment that "this is not my usual patient." With group practices, cover arrangements, and social worker duty rotas for the one on call, the case is new. Contact with an old person—swift for someone familiar—can be slow and laborious for a stranger. Moreover, the doctor encountering a person on another doctor's list does not know the relatives or neighbors usually available. Since the old person—and sometimes others too—are at risk, admission to hospital is a frequent plea at the weekend. It is simple to arrange and an easy solution for the professional people involved, although an old person seldom finds the solution as satisfactory. It takes more thought and trouble to keep the old person at home until the patient's own doctor and relations are back on the scene.

Disfigurement

Road casualties, those undergoing major surgery—particularly limb amputation, hysterectomy, and mastectomy, those with disfiguring disease or burns, vasectomy and sterilization cases, and those with loss of sight, hearing, or major functions as in strokes, are legion in our general hospitals.

If I could term each one an amputee, then each goes through the same stages of grief with regard to the lost part as one who has lost a person. The phantom limb is more frequent than the phantom spouse in such cases, and despite ingenious neurophysiological hypotheses for these phenomena, probably many can, so to speak, briefly re-create a lost limb or lost function to mitigate the loss. Even the blinded may claim he sees for short spells before finally resigning to sightlessness.

In some ways, the body loss is felt as more intensely personal than the loss of a loved one, and moreover the shame and social stigma may be greater too. Finding a new identity and assuming new functions constitute unlearning and re-learning in the physical as well as the social and psychological senses.

Doctors and nurses, justly proud of their work to limit loss and create restitution with a measure of prosthesis, meet with an apparent lack of awareness and appreciation of new possibilities on the part of the amputee. Unless the professional helpers understand when the prosthesis is out of step with the patient's stage of grief, they are likely to feel impatient with ingratitude and withhold support when it is most needed. At such times, a great advantage of the physiotherapist and occupational therapist is to provide support in these circumstances.

Separation from the Family

While we are considering the patient's grief, we should note that the grief of visiting relatives can be distressing too, for they must alter their expectations of the patient as well as empathize with his suffering. This is in addition to feelings of separation, since a spouse and children may miss the one in the hospital terribly. The accommodation of mothers in the children's wards, and children with parents, is a limited and important acknowledgment of the problem, but we are far from practicing Lambaréné-style social medicine. Provision of day rooms and interview rooms in our hospitals where relatives can spend time with patients would help; but overall, the understanding of the ward staff that the patient who is treated individually in the ward is still a family member is even more important. Ward staff talking with patients and relatives should regard such discussions as part of their work.

Parallel experiences occur in other institutions such as prisons, when consideration is given to the prisoner's losses, but the misery of the families in separation may be great. The penal system operates with callous disregard of children's needs and suffering when sometimes a distant prison is selected which makes contact between family and prisoner extremely difficult.

The argument for family accommodation in teaching hospitals is not only to encourage excellence in social medicine but because these hospitals offer regional or national specialist services, which means that families travel from great distances at times. Without accommodation, visits are few and far between and the separation experience is wretched.

Separation in the Ward

A ward patient relates not only to other people but to the routine and place, even the ward furniture. For example, it is a great comfort for them to have belongings from home in their new surroundings; soon the physical environment of the ward becomes familiar. Thereafter, transfer from an intensive-care unit (with its life-saving devices and many nurses) to a different ward (or even to a different bed in the same ward) can be very disturbing. Such bed bereavement might be avoided with different organization, or at least modified by adequate preparation of the patient for a change.

Help for the Bereaved

Help for the bereaved may lie in adopting a rather passive role like a good accoucheur at a normal delivery, since nature's course proceeds satisfactorily. Attendants keep the person company and help a bit now and then. This is the attitude which Parkes advocates. The antithesis is an active probing of the grief—in its most extreme form—an intensive flooding method. The latter, although reported in the popular press, has not been evaluated, and there is clinical evidence suggesting that forced reality testing in the early period of bereavement is likely to give rise to difficulties such as panic reaction, massive shutting out of emotion, or the repetitious reliving of traumatic experience (Parkes). In any case, for a day or two the bereaved person may require some protection from too much intrusion, but thereafter until the burial or cremation, the ritual of funeral arrangements, viewing and touching the body, visiting, the wake, funeral service, and burial, provide a good deal of probing along with the necessary social support.

It is difficult for the doctor to convey to the patient his accessibility for counsel and comfort when the patient fails to take the initiative. It is not easy for him in these circumstances, confronted by his patient's suffering, to do nothing.

How does a doctor understand that he is of value even when he may feel useless, and when his contacts with a grief-stricken person seem very unsatisfactory? I suspect that until he develop an inner voice of experience, he needs a colleague to tell him.

If the patient is not ready to talk at one time, there could be a collusion to avoid opportunities at other times as well. Prescribing tranquilizers, antidepressants, and hypnotics is commonplace and they have their value if used with discretion. However, prescribing can be a way of putting off or avoiding uncomfortable talking or expression of feelings, and prescribing night sedation can lead to dependency. Generally, drugs should be used for rest periods rather than to blanket over grief. The grief work has to be done and if shelved does not go away. Indeed, grief should be regarded as pathological only if it is delayed. Even then, the first-line treatment would be psychotherapy.

Residual grief recurs on death anniversaries, birthday anniversaries of deceased relatives, or at Christmas. Often I have had patients referred to me at these times with depression of unknown origin, suggesting that it is difficult for some doctors to recognize grief when it confronts them. Even when a doctor does recognize grief, he might realize that it should not continue beyond a satisfactory mourning period, and that a suggestion from him to this effect may enable his patient to discontinue the mourning which is no longer expected. Those bereaved people who have previously made provisions for this contingency—such as life insurance, a will, and a grave—seem less distressed. It would be macabre to have notices in the waiting room: "Have you made a will?"; "Are you insured?"; "Have you bought a grave?" Nevertheless, doctors are well advised to ask their patients if they have attended to these important matters, particularly when there has been a warning illness.

There may be a case for having psychiatrist to help doctors out with various grief experiences. I do not know how well psychiatrists perform this task, but it is true that doctors are sometimes too preoccupied with their own grief or other important considerations of a case to help the bereaved. Sometimes it is enough simply to draw attention to grief to have it recognized for what it is. Often a psychiatric diagnosis can be not only misleading but makes the staff unsure about coping. I was consulted recently about a woman in a hospital having treatment for a fractured femur. I was given the diagnosis of dementia with confusion and restlessness, and informed that she had been given very heavy sedation which had been ineffective. It turned out that her husband had died since her admittance, so that she had sustained the double loss of her husband (permanently) and her home (temporarily). When her restlessness was recognized by the ward staff as grief, they felt better able to cope, and within a few days nurses and patient could understand one another much better.

A paper by Rees (1971) probably helped a lot of doctors to realize that almost half of widows and widowers have auditory, visual, and tactile hallucinations, and illusions of the dead spouse, which can be a comfort or what Parkes calls temporary mitigation of the pangs. Otherwise, doctors may regard such hallucinations as pointing to psychiatric pathology beyond their means to cope.

References

Bourne, S. The psychological effects of stillbirths on women and their doctors. *J. R. Coll. Gen. Prac.*16:103, 1968.

Bowlby, J. *Child Care and the Growth of Love*. Harmondsworth: Pelican Books, 1953.

Caplan, G. *An Approach to Community Mental Health*. London, Tavistock, 1961.

Freud, S. *Mourning and Melancholia* Standard Edition, Vol. 14, London: Hogarth Press and the Institute of Psychoanalysis, 1917.

Hinton, J. *Dying*. Harmondsworth: Penguin Books, 1967.

Home, H. J. The concept of mind. *Int. J. Psycho-anal.*47/42, 42–49, 1966.

Kübler-Ross, E. *On Death and Dying*. London: Tavistock, 1970.

Lewis, C. S. *A Grief Observed*. London: Faber, 1961.

Lewis, E. The management of stillbirth: coping with an unreality. *Lancet*2:619, 1976.

Parkes, C. M. *Bereavement. Studies of Grief in Adult Life*. Harmondsworth: Pelican Books, 1972.

Rees, W. D. *Brit. Med. J.*4:37–41, 1971.

Robertson, J., and Joyce. *Young Children in Brief Separation*. Film Series. Concord Films Council, Nacton, Ipswich, England: 1967–1976.

10

Physical Deterioration in Patients with Advanced Cancer

Irwin H. Krakoff, M.D.

Previous discussions in this symposium have addressed the problems encountered by patients and their families in coping with the stresses of impending death. We have also considered the stresses on the medical staff of coping with the dying. Changes in attitudes during the last few years have resulted in our giving more attention to both of those areas. It seems inevitable that *concern* for the emotional needs of the dying will produce better *care* for those needs. The opening of communication which is occurring as we allow death to "come out of the closet" is helping to dispel the discomfort that doctors have felt in their impotence. As we can talk with patients, we can better understand *all* of their needs. We can discuss what may be expected to occur and how we will deal with it; in anticipating some of the problems, we can relieve some of the fears of them. We can more effectively address, also, the physical problems which may be remediable.

My role in this assembly is, I believe, as an internist and medical oncologist, to emphasize some of the things which should not be submerged in our concern for the emotional stresses of cancer.

Irwin H. Krakoff • Professor and Director, Vermont Regional Cancer Center, University of Vermont, Burlington, Vermont 05401.

There are many manifestations of physical ailment in patients with advanced cancer. As physicians we may be expected to deal with pain, anemia, infection, weight loss, effusions into the pleural and peritoneal cavities and into the pericardial space; on occasion we must deal with uremia, hypercalcemia and other metabolic abnormalities. Even when we cannot significantly prolong life, we can, with careful attention to pathophysiology, significantly relieve symptoms.

Of several important problems that could be discussed, I would like briefly to mention the problem of pain. Severe pain is common in patients with cancer. As many who deal frequently with patients with advanced cancer will appreciate, it is common for general medical and surgical house officers to use narcotics in what we would consider trivial doses. A recent study analyzed the prescription usage of narcotics by general house officers, and found that such therapy was markedly underused. We are taught as medical students that narcotics have certain side effects against which we are cautioned. With this training, when we first come into contact with patients with advanced cancer, there is a great tendency to beware of the side effects at the expense of inadequate pain control. There is great concern about narcotic addiction, which is probably overdone. Physical addiction to narcotic drugs does occur, of course, but there is a great legal and moral overlay which may adversely affect our judgment. In dealing with severe pain, the issue of addiction is largely irrelevant. Narcotics should be used as necessary to control pain. There is no legal interdiction against the adequate use of analgesics, and it is immoral *not* to use adequate drugs. If physical addiction occurs, it is just not very important in a patient with severe pain and a limited life expectancy. Furthermore, if the cause of the pain is corrected, addiction which has occurred in that setting tends to be relatively easy to treat. *Tolerance* to narcotics is a different matter; it does occur regularly with the repeated administration of narcotic drugs, and since tolerance to different pharmacologic effects of a drug may develop at differing rates, it may interfere with the physician's ability to make his patient comfortable. Possibly the most serious impediment to the proper use of analgesic drugs is ignorance of equivalent doses of different drugs, of absorption of drugs when given by different routes and of duration of effect. In a study at the Vermont Regional Cancer Center of home care of patients with advanced cancer, it was found that the dose and schedule of a narcotic prescribed even by skilled physicians in our Oncology Clinic, were often inappropriate. Adjustment of dose and schedule (most frequently the latter) by a nurse acting in consultation with the clinic-based physician achieved much better pain control than in patients who were simply handed a prescription at each clinic visit.

There are other methods of pain control. Radiotherapy to a painful osseous metastasis can provide very rapid pain relief—often without the need for protracted courses of irradiation. Modern neurosurgical techniques can often produce local analgesia without the disabling motor deficits that characterized some of the older neurosurgical approaches.

I believe that it is not mandatory for any patient with advanced cancer to suffer severe pain; we do have the ability, to a very substantial degree, to control it.

As tumors grow, they may occlude hollow organs, either by external pressure or direct invasion. It has become popular, in some circles, to condemn the use of "tubes" to relieve obstruction, on the grounds that such maneuvers deprive a patient who is certain to die, of "death with dignity." Intestinal obstruction produces abdominal pain and intractable vomiting; dying with those complications is, by no stretch of the imagination, dignified. The nasogastric tube which may appear offensive to the visitor can be an enormous relief to the patient who needs it. Similarly, tubes which carry oxygen, which supply fluids to a dehydrated patient, which prevent the sequelae of urinary incontinence, can be sources of great comfort to a patient, even if not life-saving. In our zeal to deal directly with death, we must not interdict those active measures which make life tolerable.

Coma, a frequent "terminal" event, must be analyzed. Medical and supporting staff and family members may view the onset of unconsciousness in a patient with advanced cancer as a good thing and refrain from measures which might awaken the patient. That may indeed be an appropriate position but it is necessary to be sure. Patients with brain metastases can achieve remarkable improvement from treatment with adrenal steroids and X-ray therapy to the brain. They may be restored to useful, functional existence for months. Coma due to uremia caused by ureteral obstruction may be reversed by surgical urinary diversion and that due to hypercalcemia may be reversed by radiotherapy or excision of a tumor mass which is producing parathyroid hormone. The certainty of ultimate death, a prospect which faces all living things, should not deter us from effective, shorter-term therapy.

A problem which must be dealt with in the management of patients with advanced cancer is that of resuscitating patients who suffer cardiac arrest. We now have it within our capacity technically to resuscitate many patients who only a few years ago would have been considered to have suffered irreversible cardiac arrest and death. A valid judgment needs to be made as to whether a patient is to be resuscitated or is not to be resuscitated. That judgment can only be made on the basis of an objective evaluation of what the future holds for the patient, and it is necessary to make that evaluation before the need for action arises. The emergency— almost instinctive—reaction to cardiopulmonary arrest does not allow for detailed evaluation at the bedside *at that time*, and contingency plans must be made in advance. Developing legal considerations may, in the near future, change our perception of how resuscitative decisions should be made, and by whom, but for the present, the clinician must assume the responsibility for discussing various options with patients and with next of kin and recommending a plan of action.

It should be noted that the outlook for patients with cancer is changing. Not long ago, cancer was either surgically resectable or fatal. Increasingly, we can deal successfully with systemic or recurrent cancer. Acute leukemia in children, until recently universally fatal with a median survival of less than four months, can now be cured in more than 50% of cases. The prognosis for Hodgkins disease is even better. Survival times are improving in breast cancer and testicular cancer. It is fair to state that we can *cure* a few patients with disseminated cancer, prolong survival in some and palliate all. Dr. Mount has referred in this symposium to "the legitimate aims of therapy,"a particularly apt designation. If we consciously analyze what we are doing and why, we will neither deprive our patients of useful therapy nor burden them with well-intentioned but ineffective assaults.

References

Armstrong, D., Young, L. S., Meyer, R. D., and Blevins, A. Infectious complications of neoplastic disease. *Med. Clin. North Am.*55:729, 1971.

Myers, W. P. L. An analysis of medical problems in cancer. *Med. Clin. North Am.*45:563, 1961.

Posner, J. B. Neurological complications of systemic cancer. *Med. Clin. North Am.*55:625, 1971.

11

Summary Comments

Joel Elkes, M.D.

The preceding papers and discussions reflect the cultural transformation in which we live. In an age of revolutions, one gets used to revolutions. Ours is a somewhat more complicated affair, for it reaches deep into traditions that we have taken for granted in our trade. In any age, medicine and culture are mirrors of each other, and the values of one are deeply rooted in the values of the other. Medicine's view of sickness has been a continuous conversation between the "without" and the "within," between attack and defense, between the visible and tangible causes of an illness and the less obvious and ambiguous aspects rooted in the body's competence and in the human condition. Such leads as we have in cancer involve both; and it is in this conjunction that the value of the preceding papers lie.

Essentially, we must ask the question how symbols—or the interpretation, the very perception of symbols—can injure and scar soma, and how somatic injury, defense, and healing can be related to their symbolic counterpart. These are early days yet, but clearly there must exist a relationship between the handling of information by the immune system, its handling by the nervous system

Joel Elkes • Distinguished Service Professor, Johns Hopkins University, Baltimore, Maryland 21218. Visiting Professor, McMaster University, Hamilton, Ontario L8S 4J9, Canada.

and by the system of abstraction to which we refer as our *symbolic self.* The immune system represents a marvel of self-regulatory processes, concerned with the preservation of biological identity and the evolution of the biological self. It detects the alien from "without" or the mutant rendered alien from "within." I suggest that in our symbolic life we look for cognate systems, and that "foreignness," "separateness," and "familiarity" be accepted as valid and useful in our psychological as in our somatic life. Pain indicates separation, distancing, and nonintegration; moreover, the semantic root of health is literally "wholeness." Clearly, the immune system and the nervous system are in conversation—and coping with symbols is related to coping within the soma. It is here that the endocrine system occupies a vital role in the transduction of symbolic information into somatic response.

We owe the first historic description of this transduction to Dr. Selye. Stress, as he put it, is a state manifesting in a syndrome: so deeply have these concepts sunk into our culture that every high school student knows its three phases of alarm, resistance, and exhaustion. In his remarks, Dr. Selye stressed the importance of timing, of cycle, and of rhythm in determining the responsiveness and competence of an organism. We know far too little about that.

Dr. Lewis approached the discussions as a pathologist, emphasizing the way in which mental events could affect somatic responses, including the immune response. There the role of the centrencephalic structures may be crucial, not only of the families of the older neuroregulatory compounds (such as the cholinesters, the catecholamines, and the indoles, which one might call the old aristocracy, now being superseded by a second generation of modulators, such as ATP and the prostaglandins), but even of a more important third (and more modern) generation of various small molecules, particularly the small peptide fragments, which have such precise functions in neuroendocrine regulation. These fragments may exert very powerful effects within the brain and body, making the brain an organ of internal secretion of awesome proportions and going far beyond mere electrochemical switchgear, or even a holographically governed computer.

From this physiological perspective the papers moved to social transductions with the family. Dr. Mount dealt with the cultural transformations that are taking place quietly within the medical profession. We teach more about bonding, its nature and nurture, than ever before. Death is a time during which bonds become very clear, particularly if the environment is one to enhance this quiet clarity. Environment is crucial: be it one specially conceived and constructed, or the family and the home. This type of mobilization may make events in death very meaningful and may radically alter perspectives within the family even after death.

Dr. Fulton enlarged these views. He considered the events in the smallest core group we have—the close-knit bonding of the nuclear family—and emphasized the ways in which death is viewed in our particular culture. I think something very important must have happened when man first began to bury his dead. I remember standing outside the Mt. Carmel Caves where *Homo sapiens* have lived (probably continuously) for at least 80,000 years, and where, in a grave next to a child's skeleton, archaeologists found the seeds of flowers of a kind still growing on the Carmel mountain. Can you imagine the scene of a primitive *Homo sapiens* throwing flowers after a dead child? What happens when we mourn and love as we mourn? What happened when man introduced the death prayer and the communal watch? Some supportive structures and some social apparatus emerged which, as they became important, were enshrined in our culture. I think Dr. Fulton brought out clearly one such transformation: the way in which we undergo role reversals; the way in which, in an adaptive move, we grieve anticipatorily and are then judged by society "for not grieving." In other words, the way we try to pay our bills in advance so that we may live again. It does not quite work that way all the time. The counterpoint is grieving afterward. Every culture has built in mourning work into its structure. Every religion has hallowed it. That it should now be revived, and institutionalized, and recognized in positive affirmation in our society bespeaks of the health of a society; just as its commercial exploitation conveys the regrettable converse. In such rituals, symbols become significant to the body, and verbal language remains poor facsimile of all that goes on within. Body language tells much more. Have any of us participated in a Latin funeral or an Irish wake? Feelings are there to be told, unashamedly; and in the telling there is not only telling from person to person but also from person to self.

Thus, what we talk about is *awareness*: being more aware

means being less afraid. There is, in such experiences, more room for emotional options and choices which one may not have exercised before; for more truthfulness and coming to terms with truth. We must, of course, consider what is to be told, and when, and how. And here the qualifications (and, perhaps, the rules) which Dr. Cassell brings out are cardinal. There is a relationship between truth and trust, and, moreover—as yet not mentioned—between truth, trust, and affection. Truth and trust are not synonymous. But taking them together in context, they mean affection. They come to mean the old-fashioned word of love—a very powerful biological force which, for whatever reason, we refuse to talk of in our medical culture. And yet, it is a fact that every healing profession, every religion worth its while, uses love and enhances its use. It was religious institutions, you remember, which gave birth to healing and medicine; and there is deep adaptive wisdom in the restorative healing practices which we now regard as thoroughly modern. Man is a pretty smart animal, by and large, and he would not go on adopting practices unless they served survival. If the relationship between religion and what we may call the metaphysical component in medicine is now becoming more accessible to science and scrutiny, so much the better. Coincidentally, the limits of science are beginning to expand. It is encouraging that medicine is, on the whole, reflecting a commitment not only to truth but also to trust, to caring, and to self-caring. These changes are, as yet, a small beginning, and it is only too clear to anyone who attends a meeting of the Neuroscience Symposia, or the College of Neuropsychopharmacology, that the purely somatic approach has its limitations, and that the symbolic component is far from ready for its encounter with the somatic. As somebody said, "Anyone who understands the situation is not fully informed." Let us leave it at that.

12

Telling the Truth to the Dying Patient

Eric J. Cassell, M.D., F.A.C.P.

I would like to examine the question of truth-telling in the care of the dying patient. As we know, this is a matter of some controversy (Erickson, 1974). Until just a few years ago, it was thought that telling the truth to a patient with terminal disease would do that patient harm. In the absence of a cure, it was felt that nothing could be done for such patients. Since telling the patient his diagnosis was to pronounce upon him a hopeless sentence of doom, it was therefore thought preferable to conceal his fate from him.

This view is well represented in an excellent piece of fieldwork, *Communication and Awareness in a Cancer Ward* (MacIntosh, 1977), a book which examines the question of what information patients are given on the ward of a British cancer hospital. MacIntosh found that physicians there generally did not reveal to patients their diagnosis and prognosis: they preferred to use euphemisms, such as "Well, it's an active sort of growth and it could be troublesome if we didn't treat it in the correct way . . . we're *almost* certain we've got everything. . . ."

Eric J. Cassell • Clinical Professor, Department of Public Health, The New York Hospital, Cornell University Medical College, New York, New York 10021.

The British doctors reported that they use these methods of concealment in order to prevent patients from losing hope; but I believe that such evasive maneuvers in fact accomplish precisely the opposite, and that, furthermore, they bring to bear on the patient both the stress of uncertainty and the stress of powerlessness, in addition to the stress of the illness itself.

I suggest that, in fact, these methods conceal nothing from the patient. According to MacIntosh, the patients on the British cancer ward were well aware of the gravity of their illnesses; I believe that it is through the very use of euphemisms and professions of uncertainty that patients are apprised of this. The very fact of their use signals to the patient that the subject in question is somehow too awful to speak about, a message made more ominous by the fact that even their own doctor avoids speaking about their disease directly, apparently finding it too fearful. Faced with this behavior by the doctor, the patient sees both himself and his physician as powerless and helpless. The patient has received information which tells him he is now beyond the pale, unable to act, and, in a real sense, beyond help (Davies, 1973; Abrams, 1971).

The stress of uncertainty is equally damaging. When, in an attempt not to lock his patient into an unalterably dreadful fate, the doctor professes uncertainty as to the patient's outcome, the patient—left uninformed—is at risk to his own fears and fantasies. Kafka (1948) creates in his book *The Trial* just such a terrifyingly uncertain universe for his protagonist, K. K does not know and cannot find out who his accusers are; he does not know why he is where he is, and all his attempts to find out fail utterly. This is precisely the situation created for cancer patients whose future is deliberately left vague and uncertain; they cannot be sure what will or will not happen to them, and their physician explicitly shares this uncertainty with them.

Recent surveys of physicians' attitudes toward truth-telling have shown that, in the United States, a small number never tell patients their diagnosis and prognosis, a larger number always tell their patients, but the majority indicate a flexible attitude (Gilmore, 1974; Noyes, 1973). The largest group discusses the diagnosis depending on the type of patient, patient attitude, personality, and so on. Things are changing, and truth-telling is becoming the dominant mode, partly because of our increased experience with speaking to patients has revealed that information can improve the care of patients, and in part because of the increasing interest in ethics in medicine. (That is, the demand for truth-telling is primarily a moral imperative—it is a wrong thing to lie, it is right to tell the truth.) But, as the previous conspiracy of silence often produced great harm, so, too, can carelessly revealing the bald truth.

For example, a patient of mine, a young woman who was well, moved to Minnesota; she discovered a small lump on her chest between her breasts and went to see her local physician, who removed the lesion. The pathology report was benign, but the pathologist told the physician over the phone that the last time he had seen such a lesion, it turned out to be mycosis fungoides, a lymphoma-type lesion which is usually fatal. The physician called my patient in to explain about the pathology report; he told her the lesion was benign, but that the pathologist had told him that the last one he saw like hers developed into mycosis fungoides. He then explained to her in detail about mycosis fungoides, ending with the statement, "But, we'll always be able to keep you comfortable." Within minutes, my phone in New York rang, and, discussing the visit, the woman said, "He told me more about mycosis fungoides than I ever wanted to know." It took weeks to defuse the situation. The slides were submitted to a nationally known skin pathologist, who dismissed the lesion as trivial. In those weeks, however, every mark on that woman's skin was seen by her as the harbinger of a dreadful death. And every fear was related to her life situation, the sole caretaker of two young children at the start of a new career. I had great difficulty putting the matter to rest in her mind, and, I assure you, every time a bump appears on her skin, for years, she still is going to wonder: was the pathologist right the first time?

This is an example of a kind of damaging truth-telling that is becoming more and more prevalent. We might well ask: *Did* the Minnesota physician tell the woman "the truth"? Or did he simply unburden himself of his own anxieties?

What is "the truth" in these matters? What should the patient have been told? What is the function of information in a clinical setting, and what guides can direct its use?

Is the "truth," for example, that "Mrs. Palmer has metastatic carcinoma from the bowel to the liver with evidence of continued disease activity from which she will surely die"? That collection of facts may indeed make up a "true" statement. But suppose I gave you the above information about Mrs. Palmer, and asked you, as a physician, what should be *done* for her tomorrow? Or next week? Surely, you would ask me to provide more information. The literally "true" statement about Mrs. Palmer contains almost no information on how to *act*. The statement is a diagnostic report, but one cannot *act* on it without additional information, such as who the patient is, what has been the duration, has the disease been treated or untreated, and so on.

Because information given by a doctor to a patient can do either harm or good, we must see it for what it is: a therapeutic tool, one which is always active in any doctor–patient interaction and one about which we know remarkably little. What general principles will allow us to use this therapeutic tool skillfully?

The critical issue concerns the function of information, which must be *to reduce uncertainty* and *to provide a basis for action*; these two functions are inextricably related. When this is understood, knowing what and how to inform patients becomes, if not easy, then easier.

Moment to moment, week to week, and year after year, uncertainty exists at every turn. Choices must be made, a path of action selected from among alternative directions. Whenever uncertainty exists, it is reduced by information. Whether one finds oneself in a Kafkaesque universe, or in a cancer ward, the stress of uncertainty is reduced by gathering information; first, in order to orient oneself, then to see what actions lie within the realm of possibility, then to make a selection from among those possibilities, and then to take action. Where uncertainty exists, and information is lacking, the avenues of action are limited. Where uncertainty exists, and information is unavailable from one source (for example, the physician), information will be sought from other sources (for example, the patient's Aunt Rose) to enhance the patient's potential to act in his own behalf.

Multiple sources of information exist. We generally think of the environment, the world around, as a primary information source, and so it is. If you are a patient on a cancer ward, something powerfully tells you that you do not merely have a cold. But uncertainty is reduced not only by knowledge of worldly matters of fact; it is reduced by knowledge of intent—the intent of a sentence, an act, or a person. Uncertainty raises questions of cause and effect: Why did this illness happen to me? What will happen next? The world around may not supply sufficient information; thus, other sources become important—knowledge, from whatever source, stored in memory. Unconscious or repressed needs, desires, fears, or fantasies; beliefs about how the world works, beliefs about how disease works. Other people are an important source of information; the most reliable others are not necessarily (from the physician's point of view) the most knowledgeable, but rather those (like Aunt Rose) whom the patient believes are most like him or her, or who share the same interests. When, as in the British example, a physician avoids providing information, he drives the patient into one of two equally undesirable situations: lacking information, the patient will cease to act, he will relinquish his autonomy, he will pass into a state of powerlessness; or conversely—wishing at all costs to maintain his ability to act in his own behalf—he will fill the vacuum left by his physician with Aunt Rose's ideas about treatment, his memory of how Reggie Farberg's terminal illness progressed—information gathered from any and all other sources of information available to him—and he will make his decisions according to that information.

Let us reconsider the example of the woman in Minnesota who suffered from a surfeit of information, and test what she was told according to the principles outlined above. Did the Minnesota physician who told her about mycosis fungoides reduce his patient's anxiety? No, he markedly increased it. Did he indicate, with his information, a direction for action? By no means, and further, he *made more uncertain every action in which the woman was currently engaged:* job, new life direction, child-raising, and so on. Did he increase the patient's trust in him as a physician, and promote the relationship? No, he destroyed it.

Let me stress that the patient's trust in the physician is vital to effective treatment. A few moments' reflection will show that in important situations like serious illness, there is never quite enough information to entirely eliminate uncertainty about the right thing to do, or about the future. Particularly since the information sources listed above may produce conflicting answers (which, of course, raises uncertainty even more), the patient's anxiety may be alleviated by trust in the physician. The patient, like all living persons, has a need to act, and this need is aided by the doctor's help in decision-making. When a patient trusts a doctor, he, in part, gives his uncertainty over to this physician, relinquishing it to him in trust. It follows that the doctor can fail his patient in two respects: by not providing sufficient guidance for the patient to act in his own behalf, and by not reducing uncertainty.

The question of truth-telling is now replaced by another one. What does the physician wish to accomplish with this information? Information has many facets—it has an amount, it can be spare or full. It has a kind—technical information, information about the future, information about medication. There is a degree of detail—how specific, how minute the detail to be provided. There is timing—when is information provided? It could be given at a time when a patient is unable to hear it because of his sickness or for other reasons, or it could be provided at a time too late to allow the patient to act. It has truth content—but truth content is only one aspect.

To be used properly, information must meet three tests; Does the information reduce the patient's uncertainty, now or in the future? Does the information improve the patient's ability to act in his or her own behalf, now or in the future? Does the information improve the doctor–patient relationship, which is the primary modality of treatment?

Moreover, we must recall that modern medical care requires a partnership between physician and patient. In the case of chronic illness or long-term disease, patients themselves must actively comply with treatment, from taking potent medications correctly to following dietary or exercise regimens. However, only an informed patient who feels himself a partner in the process will willingly participate fully. Thus, we must determine how much information the patient requires, what information the patient wants, and how much information is needed in order to make the patient an effective partner in his or her care.

The fundamental right of patients in such matters is to have their wishes respected (whether or not the doctor agrees with what those wishes are). Understanding patients' desires in this regard can only come about through give-and-take, through interaction occurring over time. For that reason, discussions must proceed slowly, with the doctor eliciting questions which are then answered rather than merely reciting facts.

But, it is also true that no piece of information should be imparted unless the physician is prepared to answer the questions raised by the information and teach the patient how to act against the consequences. Telling the truth necessarily raises questions: Will I be in pain? Will death come quickly? Will I be a burden to my family? Should I resign from my job or can I go back to work? And so on. If no questions are asked by the patient when common sense suggests that the information presented should raise questions, the doctor must elicit questions, or even suggest them, if necessary. The process of imparting information is not complete until all facts, possible consequences, and alternative actions have been specified to the degree that the patient desires.

I stress this point because it is also a patient's right to receive no information (if that is what he or she wants). Denial, even absolute denial, is a powerful tool the mind uses to protect the person. Where denial is present and firm, it should not be violated lightly. However, we must always be sure, when we withhold information from a patient because of denial, *whose* denial is operating: the doctor's or the patient's (Cassell, 1978).

When a physician cannot cure a fatal disease, it does not follow that he is therefore also deprived of the ability to care for his patient effectively. In terminal illness, it is not necessary for the physician to effect a cure; it *is* necessary for him or her to take action, and no set of events exists in which a physician cannot act in his patient's behalf. Technically, means exist that enable the physician to relieve most of his patient's symptoms; he or she can also act to transform the patient's initial situation of powerlessness and uncertainty in the face of illness into a workable situation, one in which the patient's autonomy is restored and preserved (Cassell, 1977). Information—passing between doctor and patient, heightened by the bond of trust, and revealed through language— is our most potent therapeutic tool toward this end.

References

Abrams, R. D. Denial and depression in the terminal cancer patient. *Psychiatr. Q.* 45:394–404, 1971.

Cassell, E. J. Autonomy and ethics in action. *New Eng. J. Med.* 297(6): August 11, 1977.

Cassell, E. J. The physician and the dying patient. In G. Usdin and J. M. Lewis (Eds.), *Textbook of Psychiatry for General Medical Practice.* New York: McGraw-Hill, 1978.

Davies, R. K., Quinlan, D. M., McKegney, F. P. *et al.* Organic factors and psychological adjustment in advanced cancer patients. *Psychosom. Med.* 35:464–471, 1973.

Erickson, R. C., and Hyerstag, B. J. The dying patient and the double-bind hypothesis. *Omega* 5:287–298, 1974.

Gilmore, A. J. J. The care and management of the dying patient in general practice. *Gen. Pract.* 213:833–842, 1974.

Kafka, F. *The Trial.* New York: Schocken Books, 1948.

MacIntosh, J. *Communication and Awareness in a Cancer Ward,* London: Croom Helm, 1977.

Noyes, R., Jr., and Travis, T. A. The care of terminally ill patients. *Arch. Int. Med.* 132:607–611, 1973.

13

The Use of Group Meetings with Cancer Patients and Their Families

Mary L. S. Vachon, R.N., M.A., W. Alan Lyall, M.D., D. Psych., Joy Rogers, R.N., Anton Formo, M.A., Karen Freedman, B. A., Jeanette Cochrane, B. A., and Stanley J. J. Freeman, M.D., D. Psych.

A diagnosis of cancer confronts the patient and his family with a major life crisis. With few exceptions, an extended period of uncertainty follows the initial treatment while all await the eventual outcome of the disease. Some authors have documented this period of uncertainty[1-3] but only a few attempts have been made to intervene in a systematic manner with groups of patients and family members to provide support and improve coping techniques during this period.[4-7] Still less systematic research has

Mary L. S. Vachon, W. Alan Lyall, Joy Rogers, Anton Formo, Karen Freedman, Jeanette Cochrane, and Stanley J. J. Freeman • Community Resources Section, Clarke Institute of Psychiatry, Toronto, Ontario M5T 1R8, Canada. Professors Vachon, Lyall, and Freeman • Department of Psychiatry, University of Toronto. Data taken from (1) "The Importance of Psychosocial Milieu in the Treatment of Cancer," funded by the Ontario Cancer Treatment and Research Foundation, Grant #298; (2) "A Preventive Intervention for the Newly Bereaved," funded by the Ontario Ministry of Health, DM #158; (3) "Coping with Cancer," supported by the Canadian Cancer Society, Toronto Unit.

been attempted with patients and family members who are living with the knowledge that the cancer is disseminated and therefore control of the disease is the best that can be hoped for.[8]

An awareness of the above factors, of the increased incidence of cancer, and of the fact that its improved life expectancy results in an extended period of uncertainty, led to a project aimed at improving the supportive services available to patients and family members in a cancer hospital. In planning such a project, it was necessary to take into account the fact that, due to the increasing number of patients, hospital staff were necessarily limited in the amount of information and support they could be expected to provide on an individual basis.

Accordingly, weekly group meetings were established in the Princess Margaret Hospital Lodge, a residential facility for patients from outside Toronto who were receiving outpatient radiotherapy treatment at the Princess Margaret Hospital. To test the hypothesis that these weekly group meetings helped to fill the above need, a research project, "The Importance of Psychosocial Milieu in the Treatment of Cancer," was initiated. This chapter discusses some aspects of this study and of other groups which emerged as an outgrowth of the initial project. Experience with the group meetings indicated that on-going support was needed by patients and families at numerous points in the illness process. To fulfill this need, group meetings have now been established for newly diagnosed patients undergoing radiotherapy treatment, patients living in the community with metastatic or recurrent disease, inpatients in a cancer hospital, parents of children with cancer, and for recently widowed women, many of whom had husbands who died of cancer.

In this chapter, we focus on four major areas:

(1) The initiation of the group meetings at Princess Margaret Lodge.

(2) Perceived lack of social support during an extended illness with cancer.

(3) The implementation of group meetings in the community.

(4) A discussion of the role of groups in the treatment of cancer.

Group Meetings at Princess Margaret Hospital Lodge

The group meetings at the Lodge were initiated five years ago at the behest of Mrs. Patricia Walker, R.N., Head Nurse. Initially, the groups were run jointly by the senior author (a psychiatric nurse) and Mrs. Walker. Now, the group meetings have become an integral part of the Lodge routine and are led by Lodge nurses who have completed the "Coping With Cancer" course to be discussed presently.

The groups are based on the premise that a time of crisis confronts individuals with potential danger and opportunity. Given sufficient support this can be a time of growth; without such support sufficient distress may compromise the response to both illness and treatment process.

The purpose of the groups are fivefold:

(1) To provide an opportunity for patients to express their feelings about their illness and thus increase the degree to which they look upon it in rational cognitive symbols instead of frightening or distorted affective images.

(2) To provide an opportunity to meet with other cancer patients in order to give and receive mutual support.

(3) To clarify misconceptions about cancer and its treatment.

(4) To meet "more experienced" patients who have lived with the disease for an extended period of time and who therefore serve as role models.

(5) To improve communication with family, friends, physicians, and hospital staff.

Naturally, the formal group meetings are not the only growth opportunity for patients in the Lodge. Its philosophy is that the time spent there should be used not only to receive radiotherapy treatment but also to gain an understanding of the disease and the problems it can create in family and social relationships. In addition to support from staff, a communal dining room and television lounges provide patients with opportunities for encounter with other patients going through a similar experience. Small informal groups form frequently and the nurses capitalize on these to get patients to share mutual concerns.

In these informal groups, as well as in the more formal ones, patients are encouraged to ask any questions they may have about their disease and its treatment. Moreover, they are encouraged to express their feelings of isolation, fear, depression, and anger. They gain understanding and support for these feelings from other patients. In addition, the "more experienced" patients are able to offer suggestions for living with the stigma of cancer, overcoming the fear of the reactions of family and friends, and coping with the panic so frequently associated with a diagnosis of cancer.

Unlike other groups for cancer patients reported in the literature,[9-11] these groups do not focus on concerns about dying. While the subject of death is openly discussed whenever it is initiated, the focus is on living with the disease and effectively coping with some of the problems it presents.

In an attempt to test the hypothesis that the experience of participating in the Lodge milieu—with its formal and informal groups—would improve the patient's adaptation to cancer, a study of women with breast cancer was undertaken. The sample and the design of this study have been described elsewhere[12] and a number of reports of the data will follow. However, a brief resumé has some relevance for the present paper.

The sample consisted of 168 women, 65 years of age and under, who were about to receive radiotherapy treatment for an initial diagnosis of breast cancer. Sixty-four Lodge patients were compared with 104 outpatients from the hospital's Outpatient Department. Stages of disease, surgical procedure, and radiotherapy treatment were similar in both groups

A number of outcome measures were used including a checklist of psychophysiological symptoms and the 30-item version of the Goldberg General Health Questionnaire (GHQ).[13] In addition there were interviews, questionnaires and case studies which supplied the usual demographic data as well as information on the subject's history as a cancer patient (first symptom, time of delay in seeking treatment, doctor's response, perceived helpfulness of various medical services, etc.), misconceptions regarding cancer, nature of social supports, and a variety of other items. A number of the items were used for purposes of comparison, throughout a series of studies on the nature of psychosocial stress being conducted by the Community Resources Section of the

Clarke Institute of Psychiatry. (Other projects include the stresses of bereavement, retirement, amputation of a limb, being an air traffic controller and being a nurse on a ward for terminal patients.) The questionnaires and interviews were administered at the beginning and end of radiotherapy as well as 6, 12, and 24 months following diagnosis. Follow-up data were obtained by mail-out questionnaires and telephone calls.

Preliminary analysis of the data suggested that the Lodge milieu was instrumental in lowering the level of distress in Lodge patients by the time they had finished their radiotherapy. The outpatient cadre did not show a similar improvement.

That this difference was due to some of the hoped-for effects of the groups and the total Lodge milieu was supported by several observations. For example, while the two groups did not differ at the time of the initial interview in the proportion of subjects who had talked frankly about their disease, significantly more Lodge subjects reported by the end of treatment that they had been able to have such a discussion. They were also more satisfied than were the outpatient group with support received from staff.

Unfortunately, the subsequent course of the Lodge patients was not as favorable and indicators of distress began to recur. It seemed clear that the supportive effects of the Lodge milieu were not sufficient to immunize the subjects against the continuing problems which many cancer patients experience. In later months, both groups frequently complained of their dissatisfaction with follow-up and particularly with the inaccessibility of staff persons to questions and to discussion of their concerns. They complained, as well, of inadequate support and understanding from family and friends and of the difficulties in coping with concomitant stresses other than their cancer. The patients who developed a recurrence of their disease were particularly emphatic about these dissatisfactions, and not surprisingly their stress levels were significantly higher than those of the other patients.

Lack of Social Support in Cancer

Data gathered in the breast cancer study about the problems of living with advanced disease were supplemented by observations from another study conducted by the authors. "A Preventive Intervention for the Newly Bereaved" is a longitudinal study of 165 women whose husbands, aged 67 and under, died respectively in one of seven hospitals in Toronto. Seventy-three of these men died of cancer and the data obtained from their widows form the basis of this section.

Standardized interviews and case studies conducted with these women one to two months following bereavement revealed that the final illnesses of their husbands produced tremendous stress. Eighty-one percent of them rated their husbands' illnesses as being "extremely" or "very" stressful. They spoke of denying the reality of their husbands' impending deaths even when told by physicians that death was inevitable.

The women wondered why they received so little help from physicians and hospital staff during the final illness. They spoke of the increasing debility which their husbands' illnesses entailed, resulting in physical and emotional strain on the women. Many whose husbands had lingering illnesses complained of the social isolation which ensued as family and friends tired of visiting and drifted away, leaving the couple to face a social death long before physical death actually occurred. Those who had dependent children had particular difficulty. Having an ill father for long periods obviously increased family tension for these healthy active children, and the mother was forced to assume the role of mediator between father and children while completely subordinating her own needs.

One month following their husbands' deaths, these women seemed to experience the summation of the stress of bereavement and the debilitating effect of the husband's terminal illness. Significantly more widows of cancer patients than widows of men who died of other causes reported feeling worse than they did at the time of the husband's death. In addition, significantly more of them saw themselves as being in poor health.

While these women had the usual difficulties adjusting to widowhood over the two years they were studied, they reported that the stress of widowhood was far less than the stress of living with cancer as a terminal illness.

Clearly, another phase of the illness, during which many patients and their families needed extra support, had been identified.

Group Meetings in the Community

Subjective impressions of the stress of living with cancer substantiated by the data obtained from the two studies led two of the authors (Vachon and Lyall) to undertake a program designed to train group leaders to function in hospital and community settings. Those chosen to participate in the Coping with Cancer course were professionals already working with cancer patients (e.g., nurses, social workers, clergy, radiotherapy technicians, etc.).

The group meetings which they initiated were not meant to be group therapy but rather were informal open-ended support groups held weekly and made available to cancer patients and their families. The intention was to develop groups for cancer patients in a variety of treatment settings, such as a cancer center, oncology units, and clinics in general hospitals, and also in various community settings.

Six ongoing groups were established in a cancer center, the Princess Margaret Hospital. Two were inpatient groups; two were in the Lodge (one structured with films and discussion, the other unstructured). There were also an outpatient radiotherapy group and a group for parents of children with cancer. Attempts to establish groups in oncology units and clinics located in general hospitals have, however, been unsuccessful to date for reasons which are not as yet quite clear.

On the other hand, the community groups held weekly at the offices of the Cancer Society have proved to be extremely successful. These "Coping with Cancer Groups" are led by professionals and attended primarily by patients and family members dealing with recurrent or advanced disease. The newly diagnosed patients who come tend to be fairly anxious people referred by physicians or hospital staff because they appear to be having more than the usual difficulty in coping with their disease.

The community groups are an important support for those who are living with cancer as a chronic illness. These patients frequently observe that they fall between the cracks of the treatment structure, since they are neither involved in active curative treatment nor terminally ill, with the problems this would entail. It is this middle group which is increasing in number and beginning to require more attention. The patients have many unanswered questions about their disease and its treatment. The groups focus on the problems of living with a life-threatening or chronic illness and the often unexamined stresses this imposes on the patient and the family, including problems with children, sexual difficulties, changes in body image, etc. In addition, patients are given suggestions about how to improve communications with their physicians in order to obtain the information they want about their disease and its treatment. The subject of death and dying is discussed insofar as the patients choose to do so, although this is not the focus of the group meetings.

As patients become sicker and are confined to home or hospital, the group leaders visit them and/or arrange for the appropriate community agencies to do so, in order to continue the process begun in the groups. Patients are helped to make the decision whether to die at home or in hospital and appropriate support is provided. Group members may visit and support one another at times of confinement but do not usually choose to do so as death approaches.

Discussion

The concept of group meetings in transitional states is not unique to the present authors but has been discussed by Parkes[16] and Schwartz.[17] This chapter represents an application of these principles to the treatment of cancer such that several crisis points in the course of the disease can be favorably affected.

The group meetings are not meant to be group therapy but are support groups led by nonpsychiatric professionals already working with cancer patients. Attendance at meetings ranges from as low as four at evening community groups to as high as 30+ in the Lodge. Average attendance is about 12. More than 2500 patients and family members attended the groups in the last year.

Groups for newly diagnosed patients focus on expression of shared feelings, meeting role models, clarifying misconceptions about the disease and its treatment, and improving communication with family, friends, and treatment personnel. These groups have a reasonably optimistic tone. They can be either structured or unstructured and are most often attended only by patients. Families seldom attend the Lodge groups because of the distance involved in traveling. Likewise, they are not often in attendance at the radiotherapy orientation meetings. This may be because patients who join the groups are more likely to be without close family members who would accompany and support them during radiotherapy.

Family members more often attend inpatient groups. Here the problems tend to be somewhat more severe. To many, hospitalization implies increased seriousness of their illness, particularly if they have managed to avoid hospitalization throughout a long course of the disease. Inpatient groups tend to focus more on "here and now" issues about treatment, how to get information from physicians, and how to function in the hospital system. Family relations and plans for discharge are not discussed as much as one might expect. This may be because patients are feeling the pressure of more immediate problems and tend to adopt a "wait and see" attitude toward their disease.

The exception to this rule is the group for parents whose children have cancer. These people seem to have a pressing need to obtain at once as much information as possible about the disease, its cause, and treatment, about negotiating the hospital system, coping with questions from the child, other family members and friends, how others have coped with the disease, and what will happen after discharge. As these parents are in and out of the hospital for long periods of time, they tend to build up their own support networks with one another.

Community groups have been quite successful. Those attending are often under considerable stress with advanced disease. Family support, while crucial during this time, is often insufficient as family members become frightened by the progressive disease. In addition, they may be under considerable stress because of the physical and emotional problems of living with a seriously ill relative. It is crucial to have back-up consultation service available to all groups but particularly so in the community groups where patients may not be in such close contact with physicians. The senior author is available to group leaders for consultation as well as referral for ongoing individual or family therapy.

Finally, as already noted, the widows of cancer patients have specific problems which merit attention. When support services are provided throughout the course of the illness, adaptation to bereavement is facilitated. But, even in the absence of such services, the availability of Community Contacts for the Widowed, a community-based widow-to-widow program developed by the authors, has been of great assistance to the widows of cancer patients.

In conclusion, it has been shown that open-ended weekly group meetings can be an effective therapeutic tool for providing information and support to cancer patients and their families at a number of points in the course of their disease. An advantage of the proposed model is the use of trained nonpsychiatric professionals as leaders of groups of patients with whom they are in daily contact. While the groups are not appropriate for every patient or family member, they have been very well received by patients and staff and seem to have provided valuable service to the more than 2500 patients and family members who have used them in the past year.

References

1. Abrams, R. The patient with cancer—his changing pattern of communication. *New Eng. J. Med.* 24:317, 1966.
2. Quint, J. Institutionalized practices of information control. *Psychiatry* 28:119, 1965.
3. Schmale, A. H. Coping reactions of the cancer patient and his family. In *Proceedings of the Fourth National Symposium. Catastrophic Illness in the Seventies*, New York, 1970.
4. Gustafson, J., Coleman, F., Dipperman, A., Whitman, H., and Hankins, R. A cancer patients' group—the problem of containment. Unpublished manuscript, 1976.
5. Vachon, M. L. S., and Lyall, W. A. L. "Applying Psychiatric Techniques to Patients with Cancer," *Hospital and Community Psychiatry* 27:582, 1976.
6. Fobair, P., Wolfson, A., Mages, N. L., Hall, J., Harrison, I., and Vose, J. Group work with cancer patients in radiation therapy. In *Psychosocial Aspects of Radiation Therapy*. New York: Columbia University Press, in press.
7. Yalom, I. D., and Greaves, C. Group therapy with the terminally ill. *Am. J. Psychiatry* 134:396, 1977.
8. Mages, N., Mendelsohn, G., and Castro, J. Concepts of Adaptation and Life Change in Cancer Patients. In *Psychosocial Aspects of Radiation Therapy*. New York: Columbia University Press, in press.

9. Corder, M., and Anders, R. Death and dying—oncology discussion group. *J. Psychiatric Nursing and Mental Health Services*12:10, 1974.
10. Franzino, M. A., Geren, J. J., and Meiman, G. L. Group discussion among the terminally ill. *Int. J. Group Psychotherapy*26:143, 1976.
11. Parsell, S., and Tagliareni, E. M. Cancer Patients Help Each Other. *Am. J. Nursing,*74:650, 1974.
12. Vachon, M. L. S., Formo, A., Cochrane, J., Lyall, W. A. L., Rogers, J., Walker, P., and Freeman, S. J. J. The effect of psychosocial milieu in the treatment of patients with cancer: A preliminary report. In *Psychosocial Aspects of Radiation Therapy.* New York: Columbia University Press, in press.
13. Goldberg, D. P. *The Detection of Psychiatric Illness by Questionnaire: A Technique for the Identification of Non-Psychotic Psychiatric Illness.* Institute of Psychiatry, Maudsley Monographs #21. London: Oxford University Press, 1972.
14. Abrams, R. *Not Alone with Cancer.* Springfield, Ill.: Charles C Thomas, 1974.
15. Weisman, A., and Worden, J. W. Psychosocial analysis of cancer deaths. *Omega*6:61, 1975.
16. Parkes, C. M. Psychosocial transitions: A field for study. *Social Science and Medicine*5:101, 1971.
17. Schwartz, M. D. Situation/transition groups: A conceptualization and review. *Am. J. Orthopsychiatry*45:744, 1975.

14

Stress, Cancer, Death—A Pediatric Perspective

Debbie Bowles, R.N., B.S.N., P.N.P. and Janet Schyving Payne, A.C.S.W.

The anticipated loss of a child through catastrophic, potentially fatal illness such as cancer is one of the greatest crises a family can experience. Cancer is now the second leading cause of death in children 1–15 years of age, exceeded only by accidents. When faced with this crisis, open communication between family, child, and health care team is crucial in alleviating stress and anxiety.

St. Jude Children's Research Hospital was established in February of 1962 and specializes in basic and clinical research into catastrophic childhood diseases, including leukemia, solid tumors, malnutrition, sickle cell anemia, muscular dystrophy, and severe infectious diseases. The health care team includes physicians, pediatric nurses practitioners, nurses, nutritionists, psychologists, social workers, and ancillary personnel. This multidisciplinary team promotes continuity of patient care.

Since the majority of patients treated for cancer at St. Jude live

Debbie Bowles and Janet Schyving Payne • St. Jude Children's Research Hospital, Memphis, Tennessee 38101. Supported by Program Project Grant CA 23099 and CORE Grant CA 21765 from National Cancer Institute and by ALSAC.

some distance from the hospital, accepting the diagnosis and treatment away from the family's normal support system (extended family, friends, clergy) is typically a time of great stress. It is also then that an effective primary care team becomes essential in forming the family's new support system so vital to the emotional survival of the family unit. Although little more than palliation could be offered to most children with cancer 20 years ago, now—with the new anti-neoplastic agents, improved surgical techniques, radiotherapy, and more effectively combined modality regimens—the prognosis for many solid tumors has greatly improved. Even when an appropriate level of realism can be instilled in the patient and family, the stress of a potentially fatal illness and its treatment can have a pronounced effect on the family's life. Consequently the basic concerns of health care professionals must extend beyond the well-being of their pediatric patients to the stabilization of as close-to-normal living among family members throughout the course of diagnosis, treatment, and recovery or death. Among the frequent problems of family members interfering with their adaptation to the stress of a seriously ill child is the denial of emotions. Mothers may be afraid to cry in front of their children; parents may avoid their feelings by concentrating on unrealistic plans for the future, or may be overwhelmed by their own shock and rendered unable to lend emotional support to one another. In this new struggle of learning to live day by day, parents often become overwhelmed with fear. They are no longer able to predict or control the survival of their child. Even when the child is doing well, it takes only a cough or slight temperature elevation, a minor ache or pain, or even a sudden alteration of temperament to panic theretofore calm parents. Also adding to the problems of many parents is a feeling of guilt. Sometimes parents feel they are being punished for past sins in their lives, or they think that their child has inherited cancer. Working fathers, absent from the hospital environment, may become forgotten grievers and inadvertently excluded from their families.

Although these mechanisms of defense and ambivalent feelings are common in the newly diagnosed patient and his or her family, it is when they extend well into treatment and begin to interfere with care of the child and functioning of the family unit that a more intensive approach is warranted. This may include counseling with the child, counseling with one or both parents, or family therapy. Utilization of the team social worker and psychologist becomes a vital part of patient care.

Much has been written about the compassionate yet frank approach to such problems, but seldom are these qualities manifested in interactions among staff, parents, and their children. The displacement of such responsibility has been a common problem among medical–nursing staff. At one extreme, the clinician may retreat from the stress of dealing with a fatally ill child to the sanctuary of the research laboratory. At the other extreme, the clinician may have become overly involved with his patients, and from a paternalistic desire to eliminate stress in the family may falsely allay their anxieties and magnify the effects of palliative treatment to the proportion of a potential cure. Eventually, the child dies, and the family—robbed of the opportunity to integrate the stress of their child's illness—cannot adapt.

When patients choose to be at home during the terminal phase of their illness, the local family physician assumes major responsibility for their physical care, and family and friends once again assume responsibility for the emotional care. However, the alternate support system (health care team) must also continue in its relationship with the family as well as assuring the family it has not been abandoned. When the child dies, whether in the home or in the hospital, the family must resume a life style where sickness and treatment are no longer the focal point. It is essential then for the health care team to be available to the family during the grief process. Many families require one or two visits with various members of the team to successfully achieve the necessary closure.

As health professionals or as family, our denial is nowhere more apparent than in our dealings with seriously ill children, because the death of a child betokens the destruction of hope. On the inpatient unit, where most of the terminal critical care is done, a rapid turnover of nursing staff is not uncommon. Providing supportive groups for nurses helps to alleviate some of the stress they experience. For the parents, it means that their aspirations and strivings for their child will not be actualized. For the professional, it means that the medical technology available was not enough and that in spite of optimal care, the life of a child was lost.

The family cannot be expected to cope with the diagnosis and treatment of cancer without some degree of suffering. However, sensitivity from the health care team can ease some of the emotional pain from this highly stressful situation.

15

Rural Cancer Death*

Stephen Nye Barton, M.D., Ph.D., David W. Coombs, Ph.D., and John P. Zakanycz

Cancer is a ubiquitous disease, a major cause of morbidity, and a leading cause of death in rural areas. Although mortality rates for cancer differ from region to region, with lower rates for many types of cancer in rural localities, the special space, time, and technological characteristics of rural areas highlight the difficulties involved in cancer therapy, research, and education. There is a shortage of doctors, pharmacists, and dentists in the rural regions of many countries. President Carter has said, "We need to reform our health care system to provide access to regular, high-quality care for our rural citizens at a cost they can afford."[1]

We know there are significant income differences between urban areas and rural areas in the United States, especially in the

*Cancer mortality data published herein were obtained through Biomedical Sciences Support Grant No. 1-505-RR7151-01 from the National Institutes of Health, Bethesda, Maryland 20014.

Stephen Nye Barton • Assistant Professor of Public Health, The University of Alabama in Birmingham, Birmingham, Alabama 35294, and President, American Rural Health Association, Birmingham, Alabama 35205. David W. Coombs • Associate Professor of Sociology, The University of Alabama, University, Alabama 35486. John P. Zakanycz • Computer Systems Analyst, The University of Alabama, University, Alabama 35486.

South. For example, in rural Alabama, the 1969 median family income was $5566 as compared to the metropolitan Alabama median income of $8352.* Moreover, rural Alabama blacks had a median family income of only $3326. By contrast, in Minnesota, metropolitan family income in 1969 was $10,771. Rural median family income there was $7488, substantially greater than in rural Alabama.

But poverty creates special problems for the rural cancer patients that go beyond medical care. To illustrate this, we can compare Minnesota to Alabama on several simple developmental dimensions. In 1970, as reported in the U.S. Census of Housing, only 71.4% of rural Alabama homes had flush toilets as compared with 90.7% for rural Minnesota homes.† However, if we look just at homes of rural Alabama blacks, only 34.3% were reported to have flush toilets. In 1970, 39.8% of rural Alabama homes did not have a telephone; moreover, more than half of rural black Alabama homes did not have a telephone. This was in sharp contrast to Minnesota where 83.4% of rural homes had telephones. In 1970, one out of five rural Alabama homes did not even have running water. Furthermore, the situation was even worse for rural blacks; in 1970, one out of every two homes inhabited by blacks did not have running water.

In addition to poverty, there are special space and time constraints that add stress dimensions to the rural cancer problem. These stresses relate to transportation inadequacies and professional isolation stemming from barriers to biomedical communication. These factors need further investigation. Before illustrating these problems, we review some geographic differences in cancer rates.

Overall cancer rates vary greatly from country to country. Silverberg reported (1968–69) relatively high male cancer rates for Luxembourg (204.6), Scotland (205.1), and Austria (191.2) with

*All income data are taken from U.S. Bureau of the Census, *U.S. Census of Population 1970: General Population Characteristics*, Final Reports PC (1) for Alabama and Minnesota (Washington, D.C.: U.S. Government Printing Office, 1973).
†Housing data are taken from U.S. Bureau of the Census, *U.S. Census of Housing*, Vol. 1, States and Small Areas (Washington, D.C.: U.S. Government Printing Office, 1973).

lower rates in Mexico (51.1), the Philippines (45.4), and the Dominican Republic (35.5). [2] The U.S. ranked 18th (153.0) of the 40 countries he listed. Canada was ranked 20th (137.8). There are regional differences within countries. Lilienfeld found that with few exceptions mortality rates (1959–1961) for most neoplasms are higher in the Northeastern and North-Central regions of the United States and are lower in the Southern sections. [3] Population density is lower in the Southeast than it is in the Northeastern and North-Central states.

Lilienfeld examined mortality as a function of urbanization; of the 31 cancer sites compared, thirteen had an urban/rural ratio of 1.33 or greater among white males; there were 21 such sites among nonwhite males. In each case the nonwhite ratio was greater than the white. [3]

Reports of rates for individual states have shown urban/rural differences. In a study of the epidemiology of cancer in Oklahoma (1956–1965) Asal and Anderson reported that nine of eleven high-rate countries were located in the northeastern part of the state and were also classified as nonrural countries. [4] Racial differences have been examined by region using trend analysis. For example, Macdonald compared two periods, 1940–1948, and 1949–1959. [5] He found non-Caucasian rates rose above rates for Caucasians in most of the U.S. Southern states in the later period (1949–1950). The deteriorating mortality position for males in general was especially true for southern non-Caucasian males; for females, non-Caucasians had higher rates than Caucasians in both periods. [5]

Haenszel[6] and Kmet[7] have emphasized the research potential of studying migrant populations. Migration appears to be a relevant stress dimension. For example, Mancuso found that age-adjusted death rates (1958–1967) for ages 35–69 among the non-white Ohio residents born in the South were 363.7 versus 180.4 for those born in Ohio (an excess of 100%). [8]

Environmental dimensions need further investigation. In August, 1977, Kuzma reported in the American Journal of Public Health that Ohio mortality rates for stomach, bladder, and all malignant neoplasms were higher for white males in counties served by surface water supplies than in counties served by ground water supplies. [9] These differences in mortality rates were not attributable to other factors known to be associated with cancer death rates including urbanization, median income, and manufacturing activity. Thus, in other places in the U.S. we might expect rural areas with ground water supplies to have lower cancer rates than areas using surface water.

As noted previously, there are marked socioeconomic differences between Minnesota and Alabama. Moreover, within these states the socioeconomic contrast along the urban/rural dimension is substantial. The University of Alabama Rural Health Clearinghouse has compared the cancer rates along the urban/rural dimension for Minnesota and Alabama. We will present some comparative data for several cancer groupings. These data show that the low-income regions earlier described as having a shortage of flush toilets, running water, and telephones have comparatively low cancer death rates. For the purpose of this report, we separated counties in both states into three categories: metropolitan, small urban, and rural. Metropolitan counties are defined as the central city counties of Standard Metropolitan Statistical Areas (SMSA), e.g., Hennepin County, Minnesota. Small urban counties are those having one or more cities between 10,000 and 49,999 population in 1970. Rural counties are those without a city of 10,000 or more population. Pooled death rates for the period 1969–71 were calculated from data supplied by the U.S. National Center for Health Statistics for each of the three county groups in both states. These rates were age-adjusted to the 1970 U.S. population. To facilitate comparisons, ratios of metropolitan to small urban and rural death rates were calculated.

Death rates for cancer of the respiratory system are highest by far in the metropolitan counties of both states. The ratio of metro death rates to both small urban and rural rates is about 1.4 to 1. When the data are broken down by race and sex, the metro/other county differences generally hold with small variations in magnitude (see Tables 1 and 2). However, there is one exception. For blacks in Alabama, respiratory cancer death rates in metropolitan and small urban counties are approximately the same. Their relation to rural rates is about 2.4 to 1 for males and 1.4 to 1 for females. Interestingly, death rates for blacks in rural Alabama, the poorest

TABLE 1. Pooled Death Rates for Cancer of the Respiratory System by Race and Sex: Metropolitan,[1] Small Urban,[2] and Rural[3] Counties in Alabama and Minnesota, 1969–1971*

County group, race, and sex	Pooled cancer death rates 1969–1971	
	Alabama	*Minnesota*
Metropolitan Counties		
White		
Male	70.2	52.4
Female	13.0	12.2
Black		
Male	49.8	119.6
Female	7.0	50.6
Small Urban Counties		
White		
Male	59.2	35.1
Female	9.5	8.7
Black		
Male	27.1	0.0
Female	8.7	0.0
Rural Counties		
White		
Male	51.0	36.0
Female	9.2	9.2
Black		
Male	20.7	0.0
Female	5.1	0.0

Source: Calculated from mortality data for 1969 through 1971 purchased from the U.S. National Center for Health Statistics of the Department of Health, Education, and Welfare, and from data in the U.S. Bureau of the Census, *U.S. Census of Population 1960: General Population Characteristics*, Final Reports for Alabama and Minnesota, *U.S. Census of Population 1970: General Population Characteristics*, Final Reports for Alabama and Minnesota (Washington, D.C., 1962 and 1972) and *Current Population Reports*, Series P-26 (Washington, D.C., 1973 and 1974).

*Rates are per 100,000 population representing three-year averages and are age-adjusted to the total U.S. population for 1970.
[1]Metropolitan counties include the central city counties of Standard Metropolitan Statistical Areas.
[2]Small urban counties contain one or more cities of 10,000 to 49,999 population.
[3]Rural counties do not contain a city of 10,000 or more population.

TABLE 2. Ratios of Respiratory System Cancer Rates in Metropolitan
Counties to Death Rates in Small Urban and Rural Counties in
Alabama and Minnesota by Race and Sex.*

Race and sex	Ratio of metro to small urban rates		Ratio of metro to rural rates	
	Alabama	*Minnesota*	*Alabama*	*Minnesota*
White				
Male	1.2	1.5	1.4	1.5
Female	1.4	1.4	1.4	1.3
Black				
Male	1.0	—	2.4	—
Female	.8	—	1.4	—

Source: Ratios were calculated from pooled, age-adjusted death rates per 100,000
population for 1969–71. Death rates were calculated from United States
mortality and census data (see Table 1 source).

*See Table 1 for definitions of metropolitan, small urban, and rural counties.

socioeconomic group in the study, are lower than for any other
category.

Curiously, in Alabama respiratory cancer death rates for
whites are much higher than for blacks in all types of counties.
However, in Minnesota, blacks in the metropolitan counties have
the highest death rates of any group in the two states. For example,
the pooled rate for black males in metropolitan Minnesota counties
is 119.6 per 100,000, as compared with a rate of 52.4 for white
Minnesota metro males.

Now let us take a look at death rates from cancer of the digestive organs and peritoneum. Overall, the pattern is similar to respiratory system cancer (see Tables 3 and 4). The ratio of metropolitan
death rates to small urban and rural rates for these cancers is about
1.2 to 1 for whites in both states. For Alabama blacks the metro/
other county ratios are somewhat greater (see Table 4).

Once again blacks in Alabama register death rates that are
generally below those for whites. We also find that the lowest
status groups—rural and small urban Alabama blacks—tend to be
at least risk from dying of these cancers. However, as with cancer
of the respiratory system, death rates for metropolitan blacks in
Minnesota are much higher than for metropolitan whites. For

TABLE 3. Pooled Death Rates for Cancer of the Digestive Organs and Peritoneum by Race and Sex: Metropolitan,[1] Small Urban,[2] and Rural[3] Counties in Alabama and Minnesota, 1969–71.*

County group, race and sex	Pooled cancer death rates 1969–71	
	Alabama	*Minnesota*
Metropolitan Counties		
White		
Male	43.9	58.8
Female	36.1	46.8
Black		
Male	47.1	110.6
Female	30.8	55.3
Small Urban Counties		
White		
Male	39.4	48.5
Female	32.6	46.0
Black		
Male	32.4	0.0
Female	24.7	0.0
Rural Counties		
White		
Male	35.5	51.9
Female	29.0	44.8
Black		
Male	35.7	0.0
Female	21.7	0.0

Source: Calculated from mortality data for 1969 through 1971 purchased from the U.S. National Center for Health Statistics of the Department of Health, Education, and Welfare, and from data in the U.S. Bureau of the Census, *U.S. Census of Population 1960: General Population Characteristics*, Final Reports for Alabama and Minnesota, *U.S. Census of Population 1970: General Population Characteristics*, Final Reports for Alabama and Minnesota (Washington, D.C., 1962 and 1972) and *Current Population Reports*, Series P-26 (Washington, D.C., 1973 and 1974).

*Rates are per 100,000 population representing three-year averages and are age-adjusted to the total U.S. population for 1970.
[1]Metropolitan counties include the central city counties of Standard Metropolitan Statistical Areas.
[2]Small urban counties contain one or more cities of 10,000 to 49,999 population.
[3]Rural counties do not contain a city of 10,000 or more population.

TABLE 4. Ratios of Digestive System Cancer Death Rates in Metropolitan
Counties to Death Rates in Small Urban and Rural Counties in Alabama
and Minnesota by Race and Sex*

Race and sex	Ratio of metro to small urban rates		Ratio of metro to rural rates	
	Alabama	*Minnesota*	*Alabama*	*Minnesota*
White				
Male	1.1	1.2	1.2	1.1
Female	1.1	1.0	1.3	1.1
Black				
Male	1.5	—	1.3	—
Female	1.3	—	1.4	—

Source: Ratios were calculated from pooled, age-adjusted death rates per 100,000
population for 1969–71. Death rates were calculated from United States
mortality and census data (see Table 3 source).

*See Table 3 for definitions of metropolitan, small urban and rural counties.

example, the metro rate in Minnesota for black males is 110.6 per
100,000 versus 58.8 for white males.

An analysis was made of cancer death rates for two other sites:
breast and urinary organs. Metropolitan to rural (and small urban)
ratios were found to be similar to those observed for respiratory
and digestive system cancers (see Tables 5 through 8).

These urban–rural differences raise the following questions:

• What stress factors contribute to the urban/rural differences
  in cancer death rates?
• What types of research investigations can reveal the genetic
  factors that predispose to cancer inducement in varying stress
  situations?
• What is the role of migration in producing cancer?
• What impact does poverty have on cancer rates?
• To what extent do low rural rates represent the inadequacy
  of rural health care delivery systems, i.e., the incomplete
  reporting or misreporting of cause of death?

Curiously, poorer countries have less reported cancer than
developed countries; and within a developed country like the U.S.,

TABLE 5. Pooled Death Rates for Breast Cancer by Race and Sex: Metropolitan,[1] Small Urban,[2] and Rural[3] Counties in Alabama and Minnesota, 1969–71*

County group, race and sex	Pooled cancer death rates 1969–71	
	Alabama	*Minnesota*
Metropolitan Counties		
White		
Male	0.3	0.2
Female	26.4	29.5
Black		
Male	0.3	0.0
Female	22.2	31.1
Small Urban Counties		
White		
Male	0.3	0.3
Female	20.2	29.5
Black		
Male	0.2	0.0
Female	15.6	0.0
Rural Counties		
White		
Male	0.3	0.4
Female	18.5	30.7
Black		
Male	0.0	0.0
Female	15.3	0.0

Source: Calculated from mortality data for 1969 through 1971 purchased from the U.S. National Center for Health Statistics of the Department of Health, Education, and Welfare, and from data in the U.S. Bureau of the Census, *U.S. Census of Population 1960: General Population Characteristics*, Final Reports for Alabama and Minnesota, *U.S. Census of Population 1970: General Population Characteristics*, Final Reports for Alabama and Minnesota (Washington, D.C., 1962 and 1972) and *Current Population Reports*, Series P–26 (Washington, D.C., 1972 and 1974).

*Rates are per 100,000 population representing three-year averages and are age-adjusted to the total U.S. population for 1970.
[1]Metropolitan counties include the central city counties of Standard Metropolitan Statistical Areas.
[2]Small urban counties contain one or more cities of 10,000 to 49,999 population.
[3]Rural counties do not contain a city of 10,000 or more population.

TABLE 6. Ratios of Breast Cancer Death Rates in Metropolitan Counties
to Death Rates in Small Urban and Rural Counties in Alabama and
Minnesota by Race and Sex*

Race and sex	Ratio of metro to small urban rates		Ratio of metro to rural rates	
	Alabama	*Minnesota*	*Alabama*	*Minnesota*
White				
Male	1.0	.7	1.0	.5
Female	1.3	1.0	1.4	1.0
Black				
Male	1.5	—	3.0	—
Female	1.4	—	1.5	—

Sources: Ratios were calculated from pooled, age-adjusted death rates per 100,000
population for 1969–71. Death rates were calculated from United States
mortality and census data (see Table 5 source).

*See Table 5 for definitions of metropolitan, small urban, and rural counties.

lower socioeconomic groups may have less cancer than higher
socioeconomic groups.

Why does race have a different impact in Minnesota as opposed to Alabama? Rates for blacks in metropolitan Minnesota are
twice as high as rates for whites, whereas, in Alabama (in contrast
to Macdonald's findings), rates for blacks are generally much lower
than for whites. More penetrating research needs to be conducted.

Although cancer death rates are higher in urban areas, the
expanded space and time dimensions in rural areas pose special
problems for the cancer patient there. A young rural black male
from the southern United States presenting with bone pain and
later being discovered to have osteogenic sarcoma provides us with
a case study highlighting the need for planning, organizing, and
strengthening health services to rural areas to insure that each
cancer patient obtains the best treatment. To provide a background
for the case study, we briefly review some general statistics about
osteogenic sarcoma.

Approximately 2000 persons die from malignant bone tumors
each year in the United States; 60% of these are osteogenic sarcoma. Moore reviewed 100 patients afflicted with this disease and
observed that 85% of patients first noted pain or swelling at the
tumor site, trauma was in the history of 33%, 5% had developmental anomalies, and 70% of the patients were dead or had metas-

TABLE 7. Pooled Death Rates from Cancer of the Urinary Organs by Race and Sex: Metropolitan,[1] Small Urban,[2] and Rural[3] Counties in Alabama and Minnesota, 1969–71*

County group, race and sex	Pooled cancer death rates 1969–71	
	Alabama	*Minnesota*
Metropolitan Counties		
White		
Male	9.0	11.0
Female	4.6	5.6
Black		
Male	6.2	6.5
Female	2.4	0.0
Small Urban Counties		
White		
Male	7.9	9.8
Female	4.1	5.0
Black		
Male	4.7	0.0
Female	3.0	0.0
Rural Counties		
White		
Male	8.4	10.6
Female	3.0	5.3
Black		
Male	5.6	0.0
Female	2.8	0.0

Source: Calculated from mortality data for 1969 through 1971 purchased from the U.S. National Center for Health Statistics of the Department of Health, Education, and Welfare, and from data in the U.S. Bureau of the Census, *U.S. Census of Population 1960: General Population Characteristics,* Final Reports for Alabama and Minnesota (Washington, D.C., 1962 and 1972) and *Current Population Reports,* Series P–26 (Washington, D.C., 1973 and 1974).

*Rates are per 100,000 population representing three year averages and are age-adjusted to the total U.S. population for 1970.
[1]Metropolitan counties include the central city counties of Standard Metropolitan Statistical Areas.
[2]Small urban counties contain one or more cities of 10,000 to 49,999 population.
[3]Rural counties do not contain a city of 10,000 or more population.

tases by 24 months.[10] Tohgo Ohmo reviewed 130 cases.[11] About three-quarters of the lesions were located at the knee joint; pain alone was the most frequent symptom (73%); the maximum diameter of the lesion ranged from 4 to 25 cm; of the 70 patients with a recorded first site of metastasis, 94.3% had the initial foci in the

TABLE 8. Ratios of Urinary Organs Cancer Death Rates in Metropolitan Counties to Death Rates in Small Urban and Rural Counties in Alabama and Minnesota by Race and Sex*

Race and sex	Ratio of metro to small urban rates		Ratio of metro to rural rates	
	Alabama	*Minnesota*	*Alabama*	*Minnesota*
White				
Male	1.1	1.1	1.1	1.0
Female	1.1	1.1	1.5	1.1
Black				
Male	1.3	—	1.1	—
Female	.8	—	.9	—

Source: Ratios were calculated from pooled, age-adjusted death rates per 100,000 population for 1969–71. Death rates were calculated from United States mortality and census data (see Table 7 source).

*See Table 7 for definitions of metropolitan, small urban, and rural counties.

lung. The actual five-year survival rate was 25.5%; patients 15 years old or younger had a lower survival rate than those over 15.

The boy in our case study lives in a rural, poor, racially mixed Alabama community in an area where the physician to population ratio is 1:7000. The 16-year-old boy is black, has a low education level, and lives with his asthmatic mother and 11 siblings. On July 2, 1975, he came to a clinic staffed by a *nurse practitioner* and complained of intermittent pain in the right leg of approximately two months duration. He stated that it hurt to put all of his weight on his right leg, and that the leg also hurt at night. He could remember no injury to his limb. No X-ray was taken. There was no X-ray machine. On physical examination no pain was elicited and there was no erythema, edema, or tenderness. He was scheduled to return.

The patient did not return to the clinic for a month. By that time, he reported to the consulting physician and the nurse practitioner that he had pain in the knee on leg straightening. He said he had limped intermittently during the previous month. On this visit, the veins of the right lower leg were prominent, edema around the knee was marked, the skin was warm to touch, and palpation of the knee elicited pain. Weight loss was 4½ lb.

He was then referred to a physician in a community 20 miles away for X-rays, diagnosis, and treatment. His temperature was found to be 100. The patient now disclosed that he had injured his right knee about three months previously while playing baseball. X-ray revealed a 5-cm lytic lesion. The patient was then referred to an orthopedic surgeon in a city about 35 miles away. The boy had no transportation, but arrangements were finally made.

An open biopsy provided a specimen for diagnosis, and on August 2, 1975, an above-the-knee amputation was performed to remove an osteogenic sarcoma. Subsequently, he was referred to another city 60 miles away for chemotherapy. However, the entire experience had frightened the patient and he dropped out of therapy. The pediatric oncologist stated that therapy was rendered impossible by the patient's reluctance to come to the large medical center.

A home visit was made by a public health nurse a year later. She noted that (1) the patient did not have a leg prosthesis; (2) the boy was not going to school; he explained that he could not afford clothes for school; (3) the patient was not receiving any follow-up treatment, and he was not receiving any form of financial assistance; (4) there was no plan for chest X-ray.

We observe in this case the stress factors introduced by geography and poverty.

Summary

The 16-year-old black boy had less opportunity for obtaining diagnosis and treatment than would have been available to an urban patient. The rural outreach clinic was staffed episodically by a nurse practitioner and infrequently by a consulting family practitioner. The clinic had no X-ray capability. The boy was poor and had no family car. The neighboring community had a small hospital but no orthopedic surgeon. The patient was referred to a larger community for amputation but there was no pediatric oncologist. Referral was made to a large metropolitan children's hospital engaged in cancer therapy and research, but the experience was frightening. At every point the patient faced delays in treatment and the final research protocol had no relevance because the boy never came to the large center once he had returned to his home community. He was unable to pursue his education. He had no leg prosthesis. No follow-up plan was instituted.

Conclusion

From an epidemiological perspective it appears that a rural person is less likely to die from cancer. The literature suggests that urbanization, industrialization, and other factors create stress that in turn promotes or induces cancer. However, further genetic and environmental research is needed. Although urban living generates stress, rural areas have stress factors, related to space and time, that influence the treatment of cancer.

Two imperatives for health policy can be deduced:

(1) More research is needed to identify stress factors operative in the urban areas that dispose to cancer.

(2) Alternative health care delivery systems utilizing technology of transportation and communication must be introduced to reduce stress on rural cancer patients.

Finally, the interaction of health and socioeconomic development needs to be more clearly specified.

References

1. *Rural Health Communications.* Presidential Edition, October 1976, Vol. II, No. 1, p. 4. University, Alabama: Clearinghouse for Rural Health Services Research, Box 6291.
2. Silverberg, E., and Holleb, A. I. Major trends in cancer: 25-year survey. CA25(1):2–8, February, 1975.
3. Lilienfeld, A. M. *Cancer in the United States.* Cambridge, Mass.: Harvard University Press, 1972, pp. 211, 215–232.
4. Asal, N. R., and Anderson, P. S., Jr. The epidemiology of cancer in Oklahoma. *South. Med. J.*68(2):193–201, 1975.
5. Macdonald, E. J. Regional patterns in mortality from cancer in the United States. *Cancer*20:617, 621, May, 1967.
6. Haenzel, W., Loveland, D. B., and Sirken, M. G. Lung cancer mortality as related to residence and smoking histories. I. White males. *J. Nat. Cancer Institute*28(4):947–1001, April, 1962.
7. Kmet, J. The role of migrant population in studies of selected cancer sites: A review. *J. Chronic Dis.*23:305–324, November, 1970.
8. Mancuso, T. F. Relation of place of birth and migration in cancer mortality in the U.S.—A study of Ohio residents (1959–1967). *J. Chronic Dis.*27:459–474, November, 1974.

9. Kuzma, R. J., Kuzma, C. M., and Buncher, C. R. Ohio drinking water source and cancer rates. *Am. J. Public Health* 67(8):725–729, August, 1977.
10. Moore, G. E., Gerner, R. E., and Brugarolas, A. Osteogenic sarcoma. *Surg. Gynecol. Obstet.* 136:359–366, March, 1973.
11. Ohmo, T., Abe, M., Tateishi, A., Kako, K., Miki, H., Sekine, K., Ueyama, H., Hasegawa, O., and Obara, K. Osteogenic sarcoma. *J. Bone J. Surgery* 57A(3):397–403, April, 1975.

16

Discussion*

Dr. *Bendich:* You mentioned that there were electron microscopic changes that one can see as a consequence of stress. Could you describe these changes please, Dr. Selye?

Dr. *Selye:* Electron microscopic changes have been described in the heart and the liver by members of my department. Dr. Milagros Salas might describe liver changes which she has observed.

Dr. *Salas:* During stress, there is an increase in autophagic vacuoles in the liver. These are the most characteristic stress changes in liver. They can be seen in the liver of intact animals stressed by various procedures: fasting, reserpine injections, large doses of cortisol injections, restraint, immersion in hot water, cold (4°C).

Dr. *Yunis:* Are there individuals who are born stress-resistant?

Dr. *Selye:* Yes. Among human beings, and certainly among animals. There are, for example, stress-susceptible pigs and they are used very much in stress experiments because if you expose them to any stressor, they will suddenly die for no apparent reason. There are genetically hypertensive rats, and if you expose them to stress they won't die from gastric ulcers or anything else. They will die from hypertension. In all animals that we have studied, it is always the weakest link in the chain

---

*This is a verbatim record of the panel discussion held by the participants in the symposium on *Cancer, stress, and death* at Montreal in 1977.

(that is, in the organ or in the animal) that breaks down. This is often genetically determined.

Dr. Krakoff: You mention, Dr. Selye, that you have had a reticulosarcoma and this is a tumor that we normally associate with a rather poor prognosis and vigorous therapy. I would like to know, first, about the tumor itself. Also the carrying out of the principle of contributing the maximum that you can during rather vigorous therapy that would normally be used in treating the tumor you describe.

Dr. Selye: It started on my thigh, and because I am given to sports—I swim everyday—I noticed it early in the form of a small nodule which turned out to be a lymph node. I immediately went to the Royal Victoria Hospital. I was examined and they said they did not know what it was. It was certainly a malignant tumor because it grew very rapidly. It did not hurt, however. It was taken out with surrounding tissue and then I got cobalt irradiation but only locally. I refused to take any chemotherapy because I thought that would be too unpleasant for me to have. I happened to be one of the lucky ones, as no other cells were touched anywhere. This was five years ago; there is no sign of recurrence. At my age of 70, I am just about as likely to die of something else.

Dr. Day: À propos of stress and cancer, I would like to raise the question about time. Stress and time relationships, particularly the biological rhythms. Would you address this topic? For example, is there any relationship in your mind between stress and cancer? Stress initiating cancer which may be expressed many years later? Is there such a relationship?

Dr. Selye: As far as chronobiology, circadian rhythms, and stress itself are concerned, one of the great experts that I know is Dr. Halberg, who is writing an article on *Stress and Circadian Variation* in a Guide which Van Nostrand Reinhold Publishing Company has asked me to write. There is enough evidence to say that there is circadian rhythm as far as stress hormones are concerned—cortisol, for instance. The problem has to be studied very carefully because individual factors play a role and some individuals are more sensitive to one factor, others to another.

Dr. Cassell: I am fascinated by what Dr. Lewis has presented. A number of years ago, I remember seeing a patient who had a cancer of the prostate. He was operated on and suffered a cardiac arrest from which he was resuscitated, but never recovered consciousness. His tumor literally grew out of his womb so that day by day the change in the size of the tumor could be seen. When he died he was a mass of tumor in the retroperineal space. I was struck by it at the time because I thought it was the model, if you wish, of a tumor unopposed by a person; not opposed solely by an act of the mind, but of the tumor unopposed by a person. And what a great many of us did or tried to do is to put the person in opposition to his disease. Our problem is that the person is not merely his immune system or his endocrine system but the whole thing put together.

Dr. Lewis: I think the point you are making is a very important one. Of necessity, we have to take a complicated interacting system that is the whole patient and his related disease and dissect it out, often in an arbitrary form, because we've got no other way. If we had a beautiful way of taking the immune system out *in vacuo*, it would be splendid; but it does not work, of course, because we know it is related to other systems, and therefore it is why I am interested in the concept of it being linked up to the higher centers.

Dr. Krakoff: I'd like to comment on Dr. Lewis's discussion. It is simply a matter of the arithmetic of the tumor cells doubling. For example, 27 doublings may produce a barely detectable tumor; 35 doublings will produce a lethal tumor. We know that starting from a single cell requires on an average 27 doublings for the tumor to become barely detectable. At this point, it is a tumor nodule about half a centimeter in diameter. Very few more doublings will rapidly increase the size of the tumor.

Dr. Lewis: I think this is a very important approach to this problem. There are also other variations. Tumors don't always grow in a homogeneous fashion. One of the points we have been interested in is the fact that sometimes tumors die off more quickly than they reproduce. This was a phenomenon that was described some years ago by a group in Australia. It is called apatosis.

Dr. Selye: I would like to make two brief remarks concerning Dr. Lewis's paper. One is that whereas there are certainly other ways the mind can act on your tumor, the one absolutely well established is that perhaps the most fundamental nonspecific symptom of reacting to stress is the mobilization of the hypothalamus–pituitary–adrenal–cortical axis which leads to an increase in corticoid production, and corticoids are generally recognized to be immunosuppressive. Now on the other hand, corticoids can also interfere with the inflammatory barricading off of metastases and thereby promote spreading. What regulates that I don't know. There is good evidence in the literature that the corticoids are not the only pathway of the relationship between the mind and tumor formation. My other remark is that an experiment such as you suggested of the tumor without the person would not be that difficult to do because there is now the so-called technique—surgical technique—of hypothalamic deafferentation. Since the nub of the whole thing is in the hypothalamus, it is possible with a circular knife—as probably many of you know—to completely isolate the hypothalamus so that no afferent impulses can go into it. That is a matter of an operation which can be done in a few minutes. If animal experiments were designed with that operation, the difference between the immunological response and tumor growths could be easily studied because they would survive indefinitely.

Dr. Brown: I would just like to comment in support on what Dr. Selye was saying: that there are many ways that the brain and the mind can influence the immune system. There are at least ten different hormonal systems that respond to stress and they respond very profoundly, and they may respond very differently to circumstances.

Dr. Luthe: I would like to comment on the slide by Dr. Balfour

Mount in which a little four-year-old girl is kissing her father on the mouth. I am disgusted and horrified by the perspective of this type of care at the point of death. It does not take any realistic consideration of what is going on in the girl's mind. You have the dying father with the head on the pillow and the little girl in the blue dress leaning over and kissing the mouth of this person, three days before death. The whole situation is recorded with precision by the brain, including the noise, the illumination, the smell of the breath, everything in detail. This is kept in the mind of that little girl for the rest of her life. Once a thing like that is in the brain you cannot erase it. Then this is going to be a major source of psychodynamic disturbance and psychosomatic disorder. I can only point toward some dimensions which I have observed many times related to exactly these types of situations. That girl will have very destructive interference for example, in the development of hetero-effective situations. Every time she will lean over a boy or a man to kiss or exchange affection, particularly when the light and illumination is somewhat similar to the one falling on the pillow, the brain will interject, and will interfere with this particular recording. Something will block the girl from really letting herself go or establishing something because this image is associated with anxiety related to the topic of death. All kinds of other material that is related to the topic of death is almost automatically hooked on and will amplify the interferences which do occur, for the rest of the life of this girl. It takes a lot of work to neutralize it. We can do it, but to my mind we have a responsibility to prevent such situations which are really not positive at all.

Dr. Mount: I fully appreciate your concern with the potential for childhood experiences to make an impact on how we find ourselves in later life. Unfortunately however, whether you like it or not, death is a part of life, and what we have to start doing is relooking at how we, and how you, look at death—what we do as a society to our perceptions about death. We don't do ourselves a favor, I would submit, by isolating that child or any other child from the realities of life that were there in the life experiences of people in an earlier generation. At the turn of the century, when most of us lived on farms (90% of us lived on farms), there was a high maternal mortality, a high perinatal mortality. Infectious diseases were commonplace. Death was seen as part of the everyday experience. It could be integrated into our concept of life. The degree to which this does not happen presently is, I think, extremely important. I just could not disagree with you more firmly. I think it is your sort of approach that has done a lot of damage. What is needed is a correcting of our societal isolation from death that has concerned Feifel and others. The risk of the little girl having harmful long-range effects following her father's death is inherent in the experience. She is suffering a significant loss. If the situation is handled calmly, with support and concern, without anxiety, and if relationships and interactions in the family are allowed to take place naturally, we feel that this inherent risk will be minimized.

Dr. Day: I don't much agree with Luthe, I regret, but there *are* features of the presentation that are troubling and *do* certainly cause stress. We have a situation of inducing stress by kindness, so to say. We live in a technocracy. Life is anything but love- and people-related. We have insulated ourselves so that we can conveniently provide death in isolation for others. I wonder about ourselves? In these hospices, we are segregating people to die. And to die in relative loneliness, away perhaps from the family and loved ones. We are a mobile society, of course, and it may not always be possible that the family *can* be present at the moment of death. For these reasons, perhaps we should identify death education as well as education for living as being worthwhile. The events of death, and leading up to death, should be shared. I have the feeling in the hospice situation that one is almost talking down to the patient? I would very much want to know how the patients respond to the physician? How do they respond to the living? Ought not the hospices to be not a dying situation? We should not, I think, segregate these people into a death situation. Rather, should we urge them to share with us a life situation?

Dr. Mount: How to respond to all those points. The first I think is the question of segregation of patients. There is a sort of precedent in this. At the turn of the century, when the thought of developing North American cancer centers came about, people thought that if you put people with malignant diseases together, that would be a negative thing. I think that the experience of M. D. Anderson, Roswell Park and Memorial Hospital, has shown us that is just not the case. Depending on how it is handled, there *is* a tremendous possibility of a patient-to-patient support system, and of relative-to-patient support—not only support by the relatives of a given patient to that patient, but to the other patients. The precedent of the cancer center, then, is one model where the grouping of people with similar problems has been supportive. In the setting of terminal disease, Saunders has shown at St. Christopher's Hospice—and I think our experience has demonstrated as well—that bringing together these patients and families allows for a quality of symptom control that just isn't possible otherwise. It allows one to bring the skills of a multidisciplinary team to the problem that is difficult to coordinate in other settings. Furthermore, what we are comparing the Hospice or Palliative Care Unit to is the acute treatment ward. I think that with time, one could develop the observation that there is no worse place for a terminally ill patient than the acute treatment ward of a hospital. From a psychological point of view, it is hard for the patient, for his family, for the other patients in that ward, and for the staff taking care of them. It has now been clearly demonstrated that it is, in fact, on the acute treatment wards that the dying are truly isolated due to the discrepancy between the goals of the institution and the needs of the patient. There is *less* isolation when a ward is provided where the goals correlate with the patients' needs; where visiting is unrestricted; where the emphasis is on psychosocial and spiritual as well as physical problems. There may be problems, I think, but the hospice approach has much to recommend it.

In terms of being, I am not sure about the implications of your comments about a "half-way technological approach." If the implication of your comment is that there is an emphasis on the affective with lesser emphasis on the cognitive, I would stress that expertise in managing these complex problems requires both cognitive skills *and* an openness to affective considerations. I feel, however, that there *does* need to be stringent quality control in palliative care, as in other forms of health care. There needs to be objective, careful observation of the impact of this type of care on these patients and on their families.

Dr. Krakoff: On the question of anticipatory grief, I think of a patient that I've seen in the last year who had a diagnosis of OAT cell cancer with a very bad prognosis; a median survival of 7 or 8 months. Almost nobody lives beyond a year. His family and his employer were well adjusted to this. His employer sent him to the Caribbean with his family as a terminal gift before he became too sick, and his family was adjusted to his impending death. But he didn't die. And after a year and a half, he was quite well but he was unemployed, the family was destroyed, the employer was annoyed that he had invested all this money in what seemed to be a phony issue, and the man himself was destroyed, although he was physically quite well!

Dr. Fulton: This is one of the problems of Keley—Orwell Keley—who's got an organization going now, a nationwide program called "Make Everyday Count." One of the things that really reorganized the cells in the mind and the emotions and the feelings and the levels of stress are just the kind of things that allow some of these talks about appropriate and inappropriate time scheduling. Glazer and Strauss and others (quite a few people) have looked at it that way, and what they are seeing is that they operate at a 5-year-old level. At the same time and side by side, they are seeing themselves operate in this odd, different way. Now they have abstractions like the fear of death, the future. It is very hard to know what's going on in the sickbed. And of course the psychology of sickness, the known psychology of sickness, is so primitive. I believe that insistent demand for information is just that. When I'm talking to patients, if it's questions I do not want to answer, I give half answers. That allows me to hear the question again, and if the same question is asked, I have to assume that the questioner *wants* an answer. I do believe, however, that I am entitled to probe. But when you talk of the *future*, uncertainty comes in. If you create uncertainty, you must put uncertainty to rest. If you create uncertainty, you must show alternative actions that may be available. To say, "Well we really don't know," or "Yes, you are dying," is no different from the situation in an adult. Its strength is different. You must always end up with less uncertainty. That is always the bottom line.

Dr. Mount: I have one problem with hearing the question twice as a determinant of what we say. It seems to me that it presupposes that we are all equal listeners. One of the interesting pieces of data from our 1973 study, examining attitudes toward death at the Royal Victoria, was the fact that of Royal Victoria Hospital physicians who thought that if they had a terminal malignant disease they would want to know the prognosis, 85% felt that their patients, in general, want to know what is going on. Of the group of Royal Victoria physicians who said that if they had a terminal disease, they would not want to know what was going on, 45% felt that their patients would want to know what was going on. In other words, how they had integrated their own finite nature and how they felt they could deal with their own fatal illness seemed to correlate well with what they heard their patients saying. So the physician who said, "You know, I never tell a patient he has cancer unless he asks me, and you know, nobody has ever asked me," tells us more about *his* inability to hear the spoken, the figurative, and the nonverbal communication than it tells us about his patients' fears.

Dr. Cassell: This research is going toward the teaching of skilled use of language, and about listening and speaking. Nonetheless, one cannot get away from the fact that a doctor and a patient are two people. A doctor is a person caring for another person. His idiosyncratic nature is part of the context. It is a mistake to think that only the doctor knows best. Usually patients know the doctors too. We do tell each other about each other. We know each other is a person by what we say. My patients whom I have had for a long time are so skilled that my own skill in dealing with them has had to quadruple. One of them said, "I knew I..." This woman had had a cardiac arrhythmia after delivery of the baby. She said, "I was in that intensive care unit and I knew the minute you came in I was in trouble." I said, "Oh, God! What, did my face look...? Did I tell you that?" "I'll tell you: You didn't crack a joke and you always crack a joke." The patient is listening too, and with good reason, because that's the most important source of information he or she has.

Dr. Luthe: I have one question that is not directly related to cancer and stress. There are research reports that in long-term transcendental meditation practitioners—as compared to short-term or nonpractitioners—there is a significant level of cholesterol in the plasma after 30 minutes of transcendental meditation as compared with controls. Would you comment?

Dr. Brown: The whole subject of prolactin and its relation to mental stages is wide open today. It was only two years ago that it was discovered that prolactin was a separate hormone in man. I can't really interpret it. But I don't find it unexpected. Prolactin is one of the most highly responsive pituitary hormones in man. Nobody has any idea of why that is so. In a variety of species, prolactin has a number of roles that are important in behavior. For instance, in salmon it is the hormone that converts salmon from being able to survive in salt water to fresh water, you see. It is very important in the migration of salmon. It's also important in the migration of birds. It's a hormone that's intimately related to behavioral aspects. What its relationship to behavior in man is is up for grabs! It's fascinating, a lead to be followed.

Dr. Lewis: I was greatly intrigued by your statements about prolactin receptors. Do I understand that there are both growth hormone and prolactin receptors on the lymphocytes?

Dr. Brown: Yes. Also glucagon. And by the way glucagon is another highly responsive stress hormone.

Dr. Lewis: Is there any evidence or is there any information regarding which subtypes of lymphocytes that these receptors are on? Because as you know, there is now a very clear awareness that there are multiple subtypes of lymphocytes which in fact interact with each other. I spoke earlier of the regulation of the immune system. This might be an area in which such an interaction could be applicable. This would be fascinating to know. If you could show that these hormones interacted with particular subvarieties of lymphocyte, that would be a tremendous way to link up the regulation of the immune system via neurohormone control.

Dr. Brown: I think that's an area that is just ripe for exploration. To my knowledge this has not been investigated.

Dr. Yunis: I know only one area. Insulin receptors are present on macrophages, on B lymphocytes and C lymphocytes.

Dr. Brown: The trouble with insulin is that it is not terribly responsive to stress.

Dr. Selye: I would like to ask one or two questions. You know when we originally formulated the concept of a pituitary shift, during stress, we had to go entirely by clinical indicators, because at that time there were no methods for determining accurately pituitary hormones. So what we saw in our rats, if they were under continuous stress for any length of time, was that the adrenals became very large, which we attributed to increased ACTH secretion. Their growth was stunted, especially if they were young. In our young growing rats, if they were lactating, their lactation stopped. In any case, male or female, gonadal activity was diminished and eventually there was a severe atrophy of ovaries and testes. So at that time, in my ignorance, I just assumed that this was due to a shift in the pituitary hormones, and that the ACTH which is most immediately needed during stress, for resistance, and for keeping alive is secreted in excess in order to permit the pituitary to produce other hormones. Now eventually, this was proven to be correct only in certain species, and only under certain circumstances, but the clinical evidence is still there both in animals and men. A lactating woman under severe stress will stop lactating. A child will stop growing. We don't need to go on but it all works out that way. Gonads will atrophy under stress. Fertility will decrease. Now I am a little puzzled by the explanation of all this because there must be some other change. Not the secretion rate, but for example, receptivity of tissues or something else?

The second question I wanted to ask was your counterposition of acute stress and depression. Now, to me the opposite of acute stress is chronic stress. Depression may be connected with chronic stress and it may not. In any case, the reactivity of depressives during stress was studied as you know by Carroll particularly, and at great length, and they have a very peculiar feedback mechanism to corticoids as have Cushing patients. I wonder whether you could tell us something about that?

Dr. Brown: With respect to the first issue, which is whether the changes observed in blood levels of hormones under stress are due to changes in release or the reactivity of tissues or the turnover: there have been a variety of studies on this. The best evidence is that there is very little change in turnover, that the primary change is a change in release. There can be some secondary changes in the receptivity itself of the cell because if a gland fails to be stimulated for a period of time, it becomes less responsive. Or if it is stimulated to excess over a period of time, it may become overly responsive and you can get adaptive changes like this. So there are changes in receptivity, but the primary changes that are seen in acute stress are in rodents and other species. There are species differences. Still the pituitary hormone seems to produce the same end result in the animal, some sort of state of adaptation. Now why is there a different kind of adaptation necessary in the primate than in the rodent? That is an unanswered question too.

Dr. Bendich: It is clear that there are a whole series of complicating and interacting factors in the various phenomena that we are discussing. But there are a number of experimental approaches to unravel some of the basic biochemistry or molecular biology which might be involved. For example, it is possible—although very difficult—to grow individual cells in tissue culture (to grow individual normal cells from humans). It is probably more difficult to grow them from humans than animals. Very often when one succeeds in doing this, they undergo a variety of spontaneous changes, such as one sees when one examines cancer cells in cultures at the same time. One can transform a cell from normal to cancer by the application of agents known to be carcinogenic in the whole human. A number of things have come about as a consequence of this and it is possible to say that perhaps this or another are the steps which are involved. But here it's possible to transform a cell to malignancy; it's also possible to observe the way the cell ages or undergoes senescence and so on, and yet this is all taking place in a simple medium without innovation, without the sort of stress reactions that one gets in a total individual. Is it valid then, to study these simple phenomena or these phenomena on a simple level? Can one really extrapolate back to the human organism? I think we haven't gone far enough with this. We've been able to observe senescence, aging, reversal of the cancer, questions that we're asking today at the cellular level. Perhaps more and more we'll come up with some fundamental answers to some of the more complicated questions.

Dr. Brown: Just further to that point, I think that what is really necessary are parallel investigations where you take the information from whole animal experiments, then look at cellular level, and do the converse, so that you can feed the information back and forth. You can't do one system in its entirety and come up with answers.

Dr. Luthe: For a while I have been concerned with attempting to answer the question whether there is a significant difference in stress reactions as far as stressor effects coming from *inside* are concerned as compared to stressor effects related to stimuli coming from *outside,* and I wonder whether the panel has anything to contribute to that question?

Dr. Yunis: I presume that one could say that stress coming from the inside could be meant by those factors involving genetic endowment which have to do with the first thing that I discussed. There are susceptibility genes of particular antigens and due to this new approach—an experimental approach in which some viruses alter an H.L.A. antigen, for instance—the mouse or man will develop specific effector cells to deal with that kind of clone of cells that have the altered antigens. But if he has a failure of that effector system, the cells proliferate and they could cause cancer or alter immunities. Under such situations, you know, that is why it is so important to consider the genetic factors. People have the susceptibility to acquire viral infections or modify their antigens according to the environment. There is an interaction between environment and genetics that would cause disease and therefore that person is going to be responding to stress in a different way than most normal people.

Dr. Cassell: If you move up from a cellular level to the organ level and then on to the social level, to nature as a whole, you see this increasing complexity, all of which follow the same kind of rules. We talk about an organism as though the organism is only man. The organism is clearly not only man. The organism is also a society which behaves in an organismic way, in a lawlike way.

Dr. Elkes: I think this question of thresholds is really rather important, and I think what Dr. Brown just mentioned is also borne out by the response patterns to psychotrophic drugs, psychoactive drugs, where the same drug, in the same dose, in the same person, will produce very different effects according to the circumstances which precede, accompany, or follow the particular medication. But what also comes to mind in the discussion of the inside or the outside being transcribed, so to speak, and encoded inside is the whole area of, shall we say, similarity, affinity congruence, isomorphism between some of the concepts which we have of the immune system, and some of the concepts which are emerging now for the way in which the brain transforms and stores information.

Dr. Luthe: I would like to touch briefly on two interrelated subjects. First, I prefer to look at stress and the area of adaptation of functions toward demands from within and demands from outside, from the perspective of the biologic principle of concordance of information. To my mind, there is a lot of evidence showing that stress increases—and adaptational possibilities decrease—as there is an increase in rupture of the biologic principle of concordance of information. I feel this is important for certain happenings at the cellular level. I also think this is important at the psychophysiologic and at the psychosomatic levels, and I also think it is very important for the management of the doctor–patient relationship in the practical situation, as Mary Vachon has just pointed out. The second point is interrelated, and this refers to observation and studies I have done during autogenic abreaction. In order to understand what autogenic abreaction is, I can make an attempt to briefly convey this.

When you are asleep and you are dreaming, it appears that certain brain mechanisms develop a programming, and that programming enters into the dream, into the contents, into the sequence of the dream. You know that Freud and others have used dreams as a valuable source of information. Now the same mechanisms that are working during dreams can be facilitated and made to work under conditions that are not related to sleep but that occur during the autogenic state. The difference is that under these circumstances, self-regulatory brain mechanisms will adopt their own programming and will give a priority to the items which are most disturbing at the mental level, in whatever area this may be, and try to reduce the disturbing potency of this mental material until the coordinating brain mechanism is satisfied. It will then go to the next point that—according to these mechanisms—needs to be, as we say, neutralized. Neutralized means reducing the potency of brain-disturbing material. Now when you watch these things, first you see that the brain mechanisms reduce, or attempt to reduce, the disturbing nature of the material that is already recorded in the brain. And much of that is related to the topic of death, particularly the death of oneself. At the same time, you can observe that these homeostatic brain mechanisms function according to the principle of concordance of information. Then when these brain mechanisms do have a chance, they will go very rapidly at any kind of material that is related to the topic of death, particularly of oneself. This may involve car accidents, cycle accidents, falling from a bal-

cony, getting hit by a stone on the head, having a hypo-
glycemic reaction, being under anesthesia, fainting spells in
church during confession, and so on. Whatever may be associated with a sudden shift, then possibility of death will be
dealt with, and the brain's way is to deal wth this in a repetitious manner; so in case there is anxiety or disturbing material
related to the death, it is important for brain to go through all
kinds of strategies that repeat the death of oneself. In the
beginning, this may be at a very symbolic level. Maybe a horde
of crocodiles are coming out of the water and are going to eat
you up. As you understand that this is a brain-directed
strategy, the best way is to let yourself be eaten up by the
crocodile and so on and so on. But the brain can repeat the
topic of one's own death perhaps 50 or 60 or 500 times and it
will do so once you give it permission. Then we see that depression, anxiety, the disturbing psychophysiological reactions, the allergies, the asthma, or whatever will progressively
be deflated and disappear. In other words, there is the progressed evidence of the revitalization and normalization at all
levels of physiologic, psychophysiologic, and mental functions.
As a matter of fact, our studies do show that with each accomplished death under these circumstances (the mental death),
there is actually a progressive improvement of the functional
situation. It is for this reason that the topic of death as far as the
biologic mechanism is concerned is very positively oriented,
because our brain, our biologic brain mechanisms, use the topic
of death in order to improve its own function. That is very important, very positive. And I think that has never been properly
viewed, and the fact that one antagonizes one's own death
may easily constitute a source of stress, and that will change
as one adopts an attitude of passive acceptance towards this
dimension permitting one's brain and oneself to adopt a pas-
sivity and let oneself die as many times as possible, until this
disturbing material has been neutralized.

Dr. Day: With these several views and studies presented, I would
like to encourage active participation in a question-and-
answer session.

Dr. Luthe: Perhaps I may start rolling the ball. From various angles it has been discussed today what to do with a patient, what to tell him, what *not* to tell him, what the patient wants to know, and what he doesn't want to know. I am left with the impression that much of this is really show business because the patient's own brain computer has all the information, knows exactly how these things came about, what the variable events and so on are that are involved in maintaining or making it worse. As a matter of fact, all the information is there and these brain mechanisms will provide you with the details of the itemized information in case you give it a chance. And when you are interacting with a patient on the ward and you are confronted with the question: "Well, what am I going to tell him?" I am left with the impression that you adopt the attitude that the patient doesn't know. I think there is a source of error. The patient's own mental computer has all the information and knows it in detail and has it all. And I think that is one of the points of departure that has to be correctly appreciated. When you tell a patient something—that he has cancer or that something of that nature is there—you are not telling anything new to the patient, because the patient's brain already knows that this is so. You are only opening a door. You're establishing a positively oriented reality situation and you are helping the patient to reestablish the basic principle of concordance of information. I think that is very important.

Dr. Day: Dr. Krakoff, would you respond?

Dr. Krakoff: I don't agree, Dr. Luthe. I think that in effect what you say is true. The patient does have all the items of information to put together to make a correct diagnosis and to interpret his own illness, but the patient is not educated, and there is so much mystique that is erroneous. Patients have not been taught to put these things together. Even a very intelligent person who has all the facts at his disposal may not arrive at the correct conclusion. I think it's implicit in the doctor–patient relationship that Dr. Cassell spoke about this morning that the physician interpret for the patient all the information the patient has in order to help him arrive at the correct conclusion. A patient cannot be expected to do so alone.

Dr. Day: Can you educate the patient? Pre-schools for example, the sexual revolution that took place 10 years ago. Sex is commonplace now. Is it feasible to educate schoolchildren to the reality of death as we know it to be?

Dr. Krakoff: Well, even schoolchildren are becoming expert in the mechanics of sex, but I think there's still a great deal that they don't know. I think there is much more that they don't know about death and the process of disease. It certainly is conceivable that one can educate people, but we have a very long, long way to go to do that, and I'm not sure that that is one of the priorities that our society should undertake. To educate people in the symptomatology that is going to add up to a diagnosis of cancer or heart disease or lupus erythematosus or hay fever.

Dr. Day: Death education ought properly *not* to be education in *disease* knowledge! Does the religious ethic of any group handle this matter, do you think?

Dr. Krakoff: Not to my knowledge.

Dr. Day: Dr. Elkes, won't you respond to this question? Does the religious ethic enter in the developing of attitudes of the patient toward the problem of death?

Dr. Elkes: I think it does if it is practiced. If it is not entirely based on dogma. In other words, I think what we are talking about is an awareness rather than a blind belief. An awareness is something very different from accepting something which somebody else tells you you should know or do. An awareness is an active process which is arrived at by the person. The question which you raise—the question of educating children, and the parallel of the sexual revolution—death so to speak is in now, isn't it, in our society? For a more general question—a much more general attitude to life and the meaning of life, and the way in which death and dying is part of living, and the parallel which Dr. Luthe drew of really reliving one's death in various symbolic ways, and thus accepting it, and thus freeing oneself, from the innominate ambiguous terror—is something which after all is done in any good psychotherapy, good experiential psychotherapy. I think the parallel which comes to mind is, say, the work which Dr. Stanislaus Gruf has done in preparing patients, and dying cancer patients, and their family for death by, in fact, a religious attitude and ceremony. The function of all religious rites and ceremonies is in allowing for an active awareness. I think the point again is as a way of *educare*, inducing education. You've got to induce and inducing has to come from within, and I think in as much as religious rites or religious practices are used to enhance an awareness, that is fine.

Dr. Day: Do they reduce stress?

Dr. Elkes: I think they are potentially very powerful coping devices. I might take the opportunity to answer your point about the age in which we live. I agree with you heartily that there is a fragmentation, that the Cartesian dualism which started after all in the old days, in the ancient religions: the places of healing were the places of religious ceremony and being with oneself through one's God in whatever form. Our fragmentation is a tragedy. But I think what I'm saying is that cultures like bodies, like healthy bodies respond, and we have now a very interesting cultural response to this alienation, and if it takes the bizarre forms of the youth cult and the whole earth catalogue, fine! But they are signs that this holistic approach is really in the making and this holistic approach may in fact be very well founded in science in the kind of data that we've heard about today.

Mrs. Vachon: Just to comment briefly on the fact that we've tried to measure some of the effect of religion on adaptation to cancer, bereavement, and staff stress. One of the things that we found in studying staff stress was that the effect of religion was very important. Now of course, this is part of the general milieu of the unit and that cannot be underestimated. However, when we looked at the effect of religion on the women with breast cancer and the widow, we found that in Toronto widows, for the most part—who may of course be different from others—did not find that their religious belief was particularly helpful to them in coping with their stressful situation. They also did not find that organized religion was particularly helpful, as embodied in the clergymen at least. We found in looking at widows that the clergy rated with physicians for not being particularly helpful. The people who turned out to be most helpful to the women in the early days' bereavement, were in fact, the funeral directors. Roughly 70% of them were rated as being very helpful compared to 47% of physicians and clergy. Over time, however, it does seem that there is some benefit from religion. This is something that we need to look at more closely. Particularly with widows and to some extent with the women who are still alive with breast cancer. Maybe it doesn't work in the early days when one might hope. Maybe one's expectations are too great and one's disappointment therefore can be very strong. But, nevertheless, maybe over time it has more of a role.

Dr. Luthe: I think that religious education is a very important factor. I find it sort of confusing to put religious education into a big basket. That really is not helpful—in case you compare an orthodox Roman Catholic education with an education of a Buddhist nature (or rather neutral without being attached to any particular Buddhist sect), and perhaps then compare it with orthodox Jewish religious education, and perhaps with somebody who didn't get any particular religious education except some historical information on who was Christ and everybody else. We did these studies and we find significant differences in reactivity. Our conclusion for the time being is something like this: As the basis and the content of religious education gets further and further away from the biologic reality of human existence, it is prone to promote more and more conflict situations and becomes a source of stress in itself and particularly in promoting conflict and anxiety situations. This to my mind is important for trying to answer and work on the question of cancer and death.

The people with orthodox religious education are actually more afraid of the second death, not of the physical death. That means ending up in Hell and burning eternally in the flames of Hell, and that constitutes a greater source of anxiety than physically passing away into the coffin. There is a decisive difference as far as stress is concerned when you compare this with a Buddhist orientation. That has practically no anxiety contact in its teachings. Then, I think there is a tremendous difference that has a significance on the outcome of the patient's behavior and the development of stress in cancer and death.

Dr. Day: I will ask you a general question. Here in Canada, you have at least two cultures, and taking into account the immigrant groups, probably a good few more. Do those of you who are Canadian physicians find a difference of attitudes in, say, the new Asian immigrant community? Are there major death attitude differences between the English-speaking and the French-speaking communities? Do they react the same? They are Canadians, but are they culturally one?

Dr. Mount: We certainly know what appears to be a significant difference between the premises, biases, and support from their faith of our Roman Catholic, frequently French-Canadian patients, as compared to our non-Catholic patients. There is a lot of cultural overlay here and there is a lot of difficulty in sifting out what are the variables. Colin Murray Parks, in his book *Bereavement,* has a very interesting table in which he tabulates the antecedent variables that may dictate outcome. Religious faith is only one of many that seem important. But certainly there seems to be a tremendous cultural variability, so that a Greek Orthodox patient has very different desires and needs than a Roman Catholic person in the next bed.

Mrs. Vachon: The Catholics in our study don't seem to be different from the Protestants. The Protestants represent 70% of our patient study group.

Dr. Yunis: In the Protestant group, has anyone tried to identify those Protestants that believe that death is absolutely a blessing? I actually have seen some friends of mine who have died of cancer and amazingly they were born-again Christians. Evangelical, very different from most other regular Protestants or Catholics because in Christianity there is a lot of fear. But have you experienced this?

Mrs. Vachon: We certainly get that to some extent. We haven't specifically tried to measure it. But we get that. We get a couple of other things. One of the things is we ask the women (whose husbands have died), throughout the course of the bereavement period whether they have any sense of closeness with their husbands, and whether they think their husbands are still some place, which is getting at a religious belief. In fact about 40–50% still continue to talk with their husbands and do think their husbands are some place, which leads some credence to the idea of a religious belief. The other thing that we look at is what we call "the silver lining question" which has to do with whether in fact you see any benefits. There it's not a religious thing, but we find that there is a blessing in that death has occurred. It's an end to suffering but it's not particularly religious.

Dr. Band: I have a comment to make to the question. I've treated cancer patients in France, in the United States, in western Canada, and now in Montreal. I have found really very little difference in the way people adjust to their illness and to the consequences of their illness provided they are informed reasonably well: first that they have cancer, and secondly what can be done to help them, whether for quality of life or prolongation of life—*and I stress provided they are informed.* In France, it wasn't the same situation. In fact, I was there as a fellow when I began my oncological career and we were warned not to mention the diagnosis of the disease. I understand from colleagues currently practicing in France that this is a very stressful situation. Most people, at least in France, don't adjust if they know their disease. They have had a lot of suicides and as a friend of mine said, "French people believe that they are immortal so we might as well leave them under this illusion."

I would comment simply on what I feel is the situation, not so much with regard to the patient but with regard to the physicians who deal or do not deal with cancer patients. It has been amply stated today that cancer carries with it a connotation that other illnesses do not have: fright, pain, hopelessness, death. Medical students who go into the medical school come with these preconceived ideas. They have seen some of their family members or friends dying of cancer and have been brought up with this mystique. They do not come neutral. We are all neutral to infectious disease or cardiovascular disease, but not toward cancer. And unfortunately during the formative years—at least until very very recently—medical students haven't been exposed to what a cancer patient is, what their problems are, what can be done for them legitimately. The curriculum stresses cardiovascular diseases, metabolic diseases, and what not. Here and there, scattered information on various types of cancer is mingled without any homogeneity. Further to that, most teachers—at least it has been my experience, and I would presume that of many people who have been to medical schools in the past 10, 15, or 20 years—have not helped in that respect. We have really learned to consider cancer patients very loosely as terminal patients. You all know how elastic that term can be in terms of time. Often comments are made that the treatment is worse than the disease and why do anything if the patient will die anyway? And in opposition to that, a lot of vigourous teaching is done in resuscitating, as we've heard from Dr. Krakoff—resuscitating people with various cardiovascular or other disease. We have learned really to fight for life and have come to also identify cancer as a death for which very little can be done. We come out of medical school very ill-equipped to face whatever the cancer patient has. As a matter of fact, I had recently a patient who phoned me to tell me that her leg was large and painful and red and I asked her "Did you consult your family physician?" "Yes, but he told me that it was a thrombophlebitis and that I should be anticoagulated and that he could do nothing for me because I had cancer." These sort of attitudes are extremely prevalent. They are at least very prevalent, I have found, in the environment in which I am working here at the moment. Where did we have to turn in order to get our education as medical oncologists or surgical oncologists? We had to turn to institutes: the Chester Beatty in England, the Institut Gustave Roussy in France, and others. This, to me, makes the problem even worse because it keeps giving the idea that to have cancer is something separate from the general path of medicine. We have to put cancer patients in institutions as we did for tuberculosis some decades ago, or like psychiatric illnesses. This has its advantages. But it has tremendous drawbacks. We keep on referring in our mind to the cancer patient as something very special; it's the leprosy of our century. And this has severed the interest of the general practitioner toward that disease. If you talk to a medical student or to a practitioner, he will know much more on relatively rare diseases like periarteritis nodosa or collagenosis, but ask him a simple question on how to handle metastatic breast cancer and he will be at a total loss.

And I must say that unfortunately in Canada the Cancer Institutions (Cancer Institutes) are also prevalent. This has brought the reflex that cancer equates to cancer clinics where the experts are. It has kept up this ignorance of physicians who should primarily deal or at least be relatively comfortable with the problems. There is absolutely no reason why physicians should feel at ease dealing with diabetes or myocardial infarct and be totally disarmed when one talks of common malignancies. What do we need? I think that we need several things in order to change these facts, let alone the terminal end of the patient. We need first to demystify cancer not only in the eyes of the public but mostly in the eyes of physicians. This will have to be done through cancer education in the medical school curriculum both at the pre- and postdoctoral level. And we will have also to consider the cancer patient globally and to develop total global expertise to support the patient from the beginning of his illness to the end of this illness. This may encompass several years of his existence or her existence where the patient will have to adapt and need various supports at the time of the diagnosis, at the time of the treatment of the primary tumor, at the time of recurrence, at the time of complications, and finally at the moment of terminal care. I would like to see personally that some study is carried out among cancer patients like the one we've heard a little earlier regarding patients with mastectomies in Toronto. That the same study be made toward the physicians who handle these patients. It would be very interesting to know what their attitudes are and how they have to some degree added stress to their patients rather than alleviated it.

Dr. Elkes: With respect to Dr. Barton's paper, I just wanted to say how delighted I am that the program moved in that direction. I think that the way in which we view the whole process of information transfer has to relative. It has to be culturally defined and delimited. By this, I support the need to include local culture, of which rural culture is an outstanding example, in such discussions as this. There is need for cultural anthropologists to move into these rural areas and describe ways of translating the information, so that it is in fact received without too much distortion or conditioning from where it is derived—the urban communities, the North, etc. This is terribly important.

17

Stress and Cancer: A Disease of Adaptation?

Paul J. Rosch, A.B., M.A., M.D., F.A.C.P.

> *What happens in the mind of man is always
> reflected in the diseases of his body.*
> —René Dubos

The concept that cancer might in some way be related to stress or other emotional factors is probably as old as the history of recorded medicine itself. Galen's treatise on tumors *De Tumoribus* notes that melancholy women (women supposedly having too much black bile—Greek *melas chole*) were much more susceptible to cancer than other females. We find a similar theme resurfacing repeatedly in medical literature, particularly in the last three centuries.

In 1701, the English physician Gendron commented on the effect of "disasters of life as occasion much trouble and grief" in the causation of cancer, and 80 years later Burrows attributed the disease to "the uneasy passions of the mind with which the patient is strongly affected for a long time." Other authors, such as Nunn in 1822, emphasized that emotional factors influenced the growth of tumors of the breast, and Stern noted that cancer of the cervix in

---

Paul J. Rosch • Chairman, American Institute of Stress, 301 Park Avenue, New York, New York 10022.

married women was more common in sensitive and frustrated individuals. In the mid-1800's, Walshe's *The Nature and Treatment of Cancer* called attention to the "influence of mental misery, sudden reverses of fortune and habitual gloomings of the temper on the disposition of carcinomatous matter. If systematic writers can be credited, these constitute the most powerful cause of the disease." Toward the end of the century, another English physician, Snow, reviewed 250 patients at the London Cancer Hospital and concluded that "the loss of a near relative was an important factor in the development of cancer of the breast and uterus."

I attach particular importance to these observations because the practice of medicine in the 18th and 19th centuries was quite likely more personalized than it is today. Physicians had to rely more upon their own understanding of the significance of the history, emotional setting, and the life style of the patient, rather than on more objective, less personalized criteria such as laboratory studies and technical procedures which characterize today's diagnostic work-up. In addition, the background and training of the physician was more apt to be heavily weighted in literature, the humanities, and philosophy, and it is quite likely that he knew the patient better and longer, knew the family, knew the nature and significance of environmental and personal background events, and had more time to spend with the patient. Thus, by virtue of his own education and orientation and personalized approach, the doctor of that time might well exhibit a greater sensitivity and awareness to this subtle relationship than is now possible in the frenetic pace of today's often superspecialized medical practice.

Lest this be misinterpreted as a denigration of the modern physician, it should be noted that in the present century, individuals from a wide spectrum of medical disciplines, utilizing a variety of more sophisticated and objective techniques, have been able to corroborate and amplify the thesis that emotional factors have an important etiologic role in the development of malignancy. Evans, a Jungian psychoanalyst, pointed out that many cancer patients lost a close emotional relation before the onset of their illness, and in the last 20 years, there has been a flurry of interest in this subject from a number of other disciplines. Using psychological tests, the distinguished British chest physician David Kissen first called attention to the fact that there were certain predominant personality traits in patients with cancer of the lung, which he characterized as being associated with an inhibition to express actual emotions. Schmale and Iker, in the United States, were able to predict cancer of the cervix with almost 75% accuracy in women who were entirely asymptomatic but who had suspicious Pap smears merely by evaluating a personality questionnaire. They concluded that this disorder occurred most often in individuals with a "helplessness-prone personality" or with a sense of hopeless frustration due to an irresolvable conflict during the preceding six months. In studies of life histories of three sets of identical twins, Greene, a hematologist at the University of Rochester, found that the twin out of each set who contracted and died of leukemia had experienced a psychological upheaval, in contradistinction to the healthy twin, who had not undergone any emotional trauma. In a 15-year study of patients with lymphoma or leukemia, Greene found that the diseases were apt to occur in a setting of emotional loss or separation which engendered feelings of anxiety, anger, sadness, or hopelessness.

Lawrence LeShan, a New York psychoanalyst, has been preoccupied with this subject for the past 20 years. Utilizing Rorschach techniques (inkblot tests), Thematic Apperception Tests, the Worthington Personal History, structured personal interviews, and interviews with close relatives of the patients, he has concluded that the most significant link in the development of a malignancy is the loss of the patient's *raison d'être* (hopelessness/helplessness)—inability on the part of the individual to express anger or resentment, a marked amount of self-dislike and distrust, and most significantly, for our purposes, loss of an important emotional relationship.

About 30 years ago, Dr. Caroline Bedell Thomas, Professor of Medicine at Johns Hopkins Hospital, commenced a psychosocial study of medical students, since they could be closely observed during their four years at medical school and, as intelligent physicians, could be relied upon to cooperate in follow-up studies for the remainder of their lives. She was initially concerned with determining what factors might be of value in predicting and preventing hypertension and coronary artery disease, and she accumulated detailed data consisting of demographic and familial factors, genetic, physiologic, psychologic, and metabolic characteristics.

Thomas was able to do this by utilizing several psychologic stress tests, a Habits of Nervous Tension Questionnaire, a Family Attitude Questionnaire, and two projective psychological tests, the Rorschach and the Figure Drawing Tests. The studies soon expanded into other areas by virtue of unexpected information which indicated possible predictable precursors for mental illness, emotional disturbance, suicide, and cancer. Dr. Thomas's data suggest that cancer tends to occur in individuals who are low-key, nonaggressive, and who do not express their emotions. Many of the individuals tended to be rather lonely persons without any close parental affiliation, or who had figuratively "lost their parent."

Novelists and poets might be expected, by virtue of their sensitivity, to appreciate such relationships. Indeed, Tolstoy's *The Death of Ivan Iliyich* bears such a theme. It was reiterated by the American poet W. H. Auden in "Miss Gee":*

> Doctor Thomas sat over his dinner
>   Though his wife was waiting to ring,
> Rolling his bread into pellets,
>   Said, "Cancer's a funny thing.
>
> Nobody knows what the cause is,
>   Though some pretend they do;
> It's like some hidden assassin
>   Waiting to strike at you.
>
> Childless women get it,
>   And men when they retire;
> It's as if there had to be some outlet
>   For their foiled creative fire."
> . . . .

Emotional loss and frustration of ambitions due to political defeat were viewed by several commentators as playing an important role in the cancers of Napoleon, Ulysses S. Grant, Robert Taft, and Hubert Humphrey.

Apart from its possible causative role in the development of cancer, stress has also been implicated in determining the rate of spread and the ultimate course of an established malignancy. All physicians have had the experience of seeing a malignant tumor spread like wildfire despite all therapeutic efforts, whereas in another patient of the same age and sex, an apparently identical malignancy behaves in a rather indolent fashion, with or without treatment. Many authors have alleged that the rate of tumor growth can be predicted based upon certain personality traits similar to those described above. One frequently quoted study done about 25 years ago by Blumberg examined two groups of cancer patients matched for age, intelligence, and the state of their cancers; all the patients knew their diagnosis. The patients were studied following their initial treatment when they were, relatively speaking, "feeling well." Those patients dying in less than two years were compared with those living for more than six years and were found to have significantly poorer outlets for emotional discharge. About ten years ago, Stavraky conducted a similar study on 204 cancer patients and concluded that the group with the most favorable outlook consisted of those who were able to show strong feelings under severe stress without loss of emotional control. Again, we encounter the feeling that "giving up" or loss of "raison d'être" may be an important factor in whether the patient survives and in determining the course of the disease. Although many of these studies would not satisfy scientific statistical criteria, they are provocative.

Nicholas Rogentine, an immunologist at the National Cancer Institute, recently reported on a group of patients who had apparently been operated on successfully for malignant melanoma, a particularly lethal form of skin cancer. He found that relapse did not occur among patients who maximized the significance of their illness, again supporting the theory that repression and denial are related to a more discouraging prognosis. His findings reinforce the value of work by LeShan, the Simontons, and others in encouraging the patient's active emotional participation as part of the management of his illness.

There are certain difficulties inherent in any attempt to prove a relationship between stress and cancer. First of all, the terms themselves are difficult to define and quantify. We all know or sense what stress is, but it is very difficult to get any unanimity of opinion on a precise definition. It is obvious that what may be damagingly stressful for one person is decidedly not for another individual. One man's meat in this instance might well be another man's poison, or more elegantly, one man's stress is another's *métier*.

It is equally difficult to equate or quantify different types of cancers. When does the malignant process start? How can its growth be accurately measured? Can malignancies such as skin cancer, tumors of the lung, colon, breast, and brain, and leukemia all be lumped together for purposes of a discussion such as ours? Similarly, what is the effect on the patient—after he has been told that he has a malignancy—in terms of altering his own personality and inducing further harmful stress? As we shall see later, it is quite likely that the *manner* in which the diagnosis and prognosis are presented may definitely influence the subsequent course of the tumor. These are only some of the variables that make it difficult to construct an experimental model that would be scientifically acceptable, but such difficulties do not preclude presenting persuasive evidence from which rational deductions may be drawn.

A masterful analysis of the multiple problems, and some possible approaches to the problem may be found in Fox's recent comprehensive analysis of the subject. One of the most intriguing and convincing clinical approaches to an understanding of the relationship between stress and illness in general is to be found in the work of Thomas Holmes, Professor of Psychiatry at the University of Washington, and his group, who identified 43 life change events and rated them according to magnitude, the criterion being how much the individual had to cope with or alter his life style as a result of the event. The following is an abridged version of how they quantified stress:

Event	Score
Death of a spouse	100
Divorce	73
Marital separation	65
Death of a close family member	63
Jail term	63
Marriage	50
Fired from job	47
Retirement	45

Event	Score
Sex difficulties	39
Death of a close friend	37
Change in number of arguments with spouse	35
Son or daughter leaves home	29
Trouble with in-laws	29
Outstanding personal achievement	28
Change in eating habits	15
Vacation	13
Traffic tickets	11

By means of a questionnaire which measures the number and types of life change events in the preceding six-month, one-year, or two-year period, it is possible to predict with some accuracy whether an individual will become ill within the next six months and, furthermore, to some extent, how serious that illness will be. The most serious type of illness is cancer. Looking at the chart, one notes that death of a spouse is considered to be the most significant life change event. The next highest event, which is more than a quarter of the way down the scale, is divorce, followed by marital separation and death of a close family member. (The first five items have been copied directly.) It is significant that those events of the greatest magnitude represent loss of a close personal relationship and far outweigh the succeeding items.

Holmes's research, indicating that death of a spouse or divorce represent the most damaging types of stress, is supported by two statistical studies dealing with cancer in females as shown in Tables 1 and 2. Table 1 shows the relationship of marital status in females in the United States to mortality from cancer of the breast, female genital organs, and other sites. Table 2 presents age-mated statistics from Great Britain which show similar findings demonstrating the validity of the non-age-mated figures in Table 1—although, again, statisticians might require more data to justify this conclusion.

The effects of stress on cancer in laboratory animals provides another source of relevant data. Workers in the school of the great Russian psychologist and physiologist Pavlov (famous for his description of the "conditioned reflex") reported that dogs subjected to severe and chronic stress had a marked increase in malignancy

TABLE 1. Cancer Mortality Rates per 100,000 Living Population of the United States
1929–1931

Marital status	Breast	Uterus	Ovary–fallopian tubes	Vulva and vagina	All other sites	Total
Single	15.0	9.0	3.3	.5	3.4	61.2
Married	24.5	35.0	4.7	.8	11.8	137.7
Divorced	29.3	57.2	6.0	1.5	81.8	175.8
Widowed	74.4	94.4	0.6	4.3	344.4	527.1

of the internal organs. Many other studies have been done in laboratory animals relating to the effects of stress on the transmission of
experimental cancer and the course of cancer in laboratory animals.
Dr. Vernon Riley and his group at the Pacific Northwest Research
Foundation in Seattle selected a strain of mice that is highly
cancer-prone, and under usual laboratory conditions, 60% of the
animals developed tumors within 8–18 months after birth. When
the research team put the mice behind a protective barrier insulat-
ing them from the normal laboratory commotion and noise—which
conceivably could generate anxiety and stress—only 7% of the
mice developed cancer during a 14-month period. Conversely, a
separate experiment showed that simply rotating the animals
gently on a turntable was sufficient to promote significantly higher
cancer rates. Another study done at Stanford University School of
Medicine dealt with the effects of stress on virus-induced tumors in
mice. The maximum tumor size was increased by three days of
electric shock stress following the virus inoculation, and it was also
noted that female mice spontaneously displaying fighting or an-
tagonistic behavior developed smaller tumors. However, there
may also be certain adaptive responses to stress which are helpful,

TABLE 2. Death Rates per 100,000 Living, All Forms of Cancer, England and Wales,
1930–1932

Marital status	Age 25	Age 35	Age 45	Age 55	Age 65	Age 70 and over
Spinsters	126 ± 0.6	68 ± 2.0	219 ± 4.1	416 ± 6.7	635 ± 13.1	961 ± 14.5
Married	169 ± 0.5	75.1 ± 2.0	202 ± 1.0	401 ± 3.3	639 ± 8.1	962 ± 11.2
Widowed and Divorced	161 ± 3.6	89 ± 3.9	246 ± 5.1	432 ± 5.1	692 ± 9.3	1084 ± 7.8

and in other experiments a *reduction* in tumor size was noted in females that were shocked for three days *prior* to virus inoculation. Another study done at Howard University also showed that behavioral stress could be utilized to inhibit the growth and development of transplanted and induced tumors in rats. This type of activity is seen to correspond best to that phase of Professor Selye's general adaptation syndrome known as the "stage of resistance," wherein body defenses are enhanced, and leads us to a consideration of the physiologic mechanisms whereby stress might cause cancer.

A wide range of substances and factors have been implicated in the cause of a variety of cancers. They include irradiation, and cell irritants of a physical or chemical nature, such as asbestos, coal tar, and excessive local heat. However, the two most important agencies which have been shown to exert an influence on the development and subsequent course of malignancy are hormonal activity and the immunologic status of the individual. It is also likely that the central nervous system plays a significant role in the mediation of these important influences. It is therefore, most pertinent to appreciate that these body activities are the most susceptible to the effects of stress, and, indeed, are used as criteria to monitor and characterize the effects of stress in humans.

The hormonal and central nervous system effects of acute stress, with respect to the release of adrenalin and stimulation of the sympathetic nervous system, were first clearly expounded by the great physiologist Walter Cannon in the early 1920's. They were subsequently expanded by the extensive investigations of Selye at the University of Montreal, who demonstrated the role of the pituitary and adrenal cortex in what he termed the "alarm reaction." In recent years, the work of John Mason at the Walter Reed Army Institute of Research (now at Yale University) and others has indicated the participation of other pituitary hormones in this response, notably prolactin (the growth hormone) and agents influencing thyroid and sexual function. Other studies on the release of neurohumoral agents in the brain and newer work on the prostaglandins will undoubtedly further enlarge the scope of hormonal participation and mediation of the response to stress.

We read daily about the possible role of hormones as causative factors in cancer of the breast and uterus. The use of various sex hormones to treat these lesions and cancer of the prostate are well known. Studies of estrogen receptor activity are now performed routinely on breast cancer tissue removed at surgery to determine the appropriateness of hormonal manipulation as a mode of treatment. Similarly, removal of certain hormone-forming organs is also utilized in the management of a variety of malignancies. Other adrenal-cortical type hormones such as cortisone are also employed in many chemotherapeutic programs. It is clear that the major effects of stress are demonstrated by changes in hormonal activity and, on the other hand, changes in hormonal activity have powerful influences on the malignant process, thus completing that link.

One of the current theories of how cancer starts states that tumor cells of a malignant nature are constantly present through our system. In susceptible individuals, such cells are able to implant themselves and multiply into malignant lesions, while other persons exhibit a natural resistance to such implantation. This may have to do with the body's ability to recognize and destroy these cells—a function of the immune system. When the organism is exposed to a foreign agent like a virus (measles, hepatitis, polio), it responds by manufacturing antibodies, which have the specific property of combatting or increasing resistance to the offending agent. That is why it is rare to have more than one attack of such virus infections as German measles. This property is exploited as the basis of various immunization techniques in which the susceptible patient is exposed to an attenuated form of the virus, to which he then reacts by creating sufficient defenses through his immune system to thwart a subsequent infection by the same or similar agents. For instance, the eradication of smallpox came about through the observation that by vaccinating children with small amounts of the cowpox virus (which produces only a slight local reaction in man), this initial exposure would stimulate the formation of antibodies to the closely related—but much more virulent and deadly—smallpox virus.

Conversely, loss of the body's immune mechanism is associated with an increased susceptibility to, and rapid spread of, infectious processes. The herpes simplex virus, which is apparently constantly present in the cell, is usually quiescent; but when resistance is lowered, clinical appearance is manifested as sores about the lips and mucous membranes of the mouth. These lesions are commonly referred to as "cold sores" or "fever blisters," implying that they occur during periods of lowered resistance. It is also of interest to note that the clinical appearance of two closely related viruses are linked with cancer. Patients with herpes zoster infection (commonly known as shingles) are thought to exhibit diminished immunologic defenses and have a higher incidence of cancer. Herpes simplex II virus, which is responsible for recurrent genital lesions, is said to predispose to cervical cancer.

Similarly, adrenal-cortical hormones interfere with the body's immune system or ability to make antibodies, and this property is used clinically to prevent rejection of organ transplants and grafts that the body perceives as foreign. When cortisone was first made available, it was noted that many patients who received it for chronic disorders such as rheumatoid arthritis suffered a reactivation of previously quiescent tuberculosis, presumably due to inhibition of a previously effective defense mechanism. The effect of cortisone and other similar adrenal-cortical-type hormones are clinically recognized as causing a rapid spread of bacterial and viral infections and are generally contraindicated in infection because of this.

Selye's research clearly demonstrated that stimulation of the adrenal cortex was the hallmark of the organism's response to acute stress, and that as part of this "alarm reaction" there was also a marked involution of lymphatic tissue and of the thymus, the major gland of the immune system. Thus, acute stress obviously could cause loss of immune protection.

Psychologists Klaus and Marjorie Bahnson of the Eastern Pennsylvania Psychological Institute have found a strong correlation between depression and decreased immunologic capacity. More recently, workers in Sydney, Australia showed that loss of a spouse was accompanied by marked reduction in immune function two to six weeks after the event, and that this impairment occurred apart from any apparent significant change in hormonal activity, suggesting that such a response may be mediated directly and not require adrenal-cortical participation. Other evidence suggests that interferon—a nonspecific polypeptide which is one of the basic defenses against virus infections—is also suppressed under conditions of emotional stress.

Thus far, we have reviewed evidence suggesting a strong relationship between certain emotional states such as depression, particularly bereavement or loss of a strong emotional relationship, and subsequent development of malignancy.We have also noted that such factors represent the most potent cause of stress for humans. Studies with laboratory animals similarly show a strong relationship between stress and experimental cancer. It is apparent that the physiologic effects of stress are reflected in the endocrine system and in the immunologic defense mechanism of the body, and that these are probably two of the most important factors in determining susceptibility and resistance to malignant growth. How does this relate to cancer as a "disease of adaptation" and what is meant by this term?

During the latter half of the nineteenth century, the great French physiologist Claude Bernard promulgated the theory that one of the most characteristic features of living organisms is their apparent ability to maintain the constancy of the internal environment (*milieu intérieur*) despite dramatic changes in environmental surroundings. By internal environment, Bernard meant the physical and chemical composition of the fluids that surround the cells of the body. Thus, although the organism might consume large amounts of certain chemicals such as salt, and though the atmospheric conditions might vary, certain adaptive mechanisms came into play designed to preserve the status quo. We all know that regardless of the temperature outside—whether it be 120°F or 20°F—the body temperature tends to remain at 98.6°F as a function of complex adaptive responses. Similarly, when large amounts of sugar are consumed, temporary changes in the concentration of this substance in the blood occur, but various physiologic responses involving the pituitary, adrenals, pancreas, and kidneys rapidly restore blood sugar levels to normal. Loss of such adaptational responses implies illness and portends death.

In the early part of this century, these theories were expanded at Harvard by Walter Cannon, who termed this power to maintain the integrity of the internal environment *homeostasis,* or the *steady state.* Cannon described the changes which occurred when the organism was severely threatened, indicating that the resultant stimulation of the sympathetic nervous system and release of adrenalin was purposeful and designed to prepare the animal for "fight or flight." The action of adrenalin caused a release of energy stored in the liver with a resultant rise in the blood sugar to provide more fuel for active cells, an increase in the heart rate and a dilatation of blood vessels in critical areas to increase the availability of nutrients and oxygen, a decrease in the coagulability of the blood to minimize hemorrhage, and an increased efficiency of muscular contraction. The pupils dilated to improve vision and a host of other phenomena ensued designed to satisfy functional needs and improve or enhance existing capabilities.

Bernard and Cannon provided the background for the brilliant and revolutionary theories of Hans Selye, who began studying the effects of stress in laboratory animals over 40 years ago. Using a profusion of techniques that embraced biochemistry, steroid chemistry, physiology, experimental surgery, anatomic and microscopic pathology, he carefully delineated the nature of the animal's response to acute stress which he termed the "alarm reaction." This involved marked activation of the pituitary–adrenal axis with the release of hormones such as ACTH and cortisone, marked shrinkage of the thymus and other lymphoid tissues, as well as acute gastric ulcerations. Exposure to prolonged stress resulted in a "stage of resistance," during which the organism's ability to resist the effects of the stressor were enhanced. And finally, if the stress persisted, there ensued a "stage of exhaustion," wherein adaptive and reparative mechanisms gave out. A variety of illnesses followed, or death occurred. This tripartite response, which appeared to be nonspecific and could be induced by a variety of noxious agents, was termed by Selye the "general adaptation syndrome." Discovery that certain disorders such as hypertension, arthritis, and peptic ulcers could be produced in the laboratory as a consequence of stress led to the concept of these illnesses as being "diseases of adaptation."

Implicit in Cannon's and Selye's theories, and most important for our thesis, is the teleologic premise that biologic responses to stress may have had some purposeful significance in primitive times or in lower forms of life but in higher stages have become inappropriate, and can indeed prove harmful or even fatal. Some of these responses seem useless or superfluous, such as the bristling of the hair on the back of the neck as a concomitant of fear; but on careful reflection, one can see that this mechanism makes the frightened cat seem fiercer, or that stimulation of these same arrector pili muscles provides a vital means of defense for the porcupine. We must also remember that nature often hyperreacts to a stimulus or need by responses that are exaggerated—for instance, the occasional development of disfiguring keloids in scar formation, or the local response to excessive heat as with clay pipe smokers in whom malignancy occurs at the site of injured tissue attempting to repair itself.

A similar phenomenon occurs in evolution. In a previous review of this subject, I have referred to the principle of *opportunism* in evolution, which is best defined as responding to or fulfilling a need with whatever means are available, even if they are not the optimal means or may ultimately prove harmful. In that essay, written over 20 years ago, I used as an example the variation in the development of horns by some 23 species of antelope in the Belgian Congo [now Zaïre]. The marked differences in anatomical configuration and functional effect do not seem to serve any rational purpose, and in some instances are perhaps disadvantageous and prohibitively unwieldy (as in the kudu). In rewriting that article today, I should choose the development of malignancy in man to illustrate this very point.

As one descends the phylogenetic scale and examines lower forms of life, it becomes apparent that the incidence of cancer progressively decreases. Conversely, the ability of the organism to regenerate tissue, organs, or even parts of the body increases proportionately. Among simpler organisms, certain types of invertebrates have the ability to sever parts of their anatomy when irritated; obviously, this capacity has survival value only if the animal possesses an equally remarkable ability to regenerate the cast-off portion from the available cell remnants. The starfish can grow a new appendage and the newt can regenerate its tail. Human beings, however, do not have such regenerative powers. I should like to suggest that the human cancer chromosome—or whatever else one chooses to call it (genome, DNA molecule, or virus)—is the modern vestige or replica of this regenerative trait which was once vital to the organism's survival and adaptation but now has actually become dangerous to it. Thus, although the primitive cellular response to loss, injury, or irritation is purposeful new growth or regeneration, this capability is not preserved in man, in whom this response can appear as new growth or neoplasia with far more sinister consequences.

To support such an hypothesis, let me point out that recent experiments have shown that if one injects into the limb of a newt chemicals which are known to result in the development of cancer in man, malignancy does not occur. Instead, the newt grows an accessory limb. If the lens of the eye of this animal is removed surgically and similar carcinogenic agents are implanted, again there is no resultant cancer, but instead a new lens is regenerated. In other words, the same stimulus apparently induces either regeneration or malignancy, depending upon the organism's stage of evolution.

Additional corroboration may be found in a recent article in the *New England Journal of Medicine* that has attracted much publicity and which refers to the phenomenon of the "born-again spleen." The authors reported a series of cases of rupture of the spleen in which, although the spleen had been removed surgically, remnants of functioning splenic tissue could be demonstrated many years later, suggesting for the first time that successful regeneration of an organ could occur spontaneously in humans. Apparently, splenic tissue has this capacity, and presumably the regenerative mechanism in this organ does function purposefully. It is therefore not surprising to learn that the spleen is also unique in that is the only organ in humans that does not give rise to primary cancer! It is also interesting to note that accessory spleens—spleniculi—are not uncommon. In very rare cases, several hundred have been present, representing a reversion to a primitive condition in which splenic tissue is not localized in a definite organ but scattered throughout the gastrointestinal tract, so that from the standpoint of comparative anatomy, the spleen retains certain vestigial characteristics from which it may derive such potential.

The leap from physical to emotional loss should not be troublesome, since even in lower forms of life the ability to regenerate tissues must involve something more than a simple local response and include, through some systemic humoral or nervous system pathway, participation of the organism as a whole. The phenomenon of loss is quite likely appreciated by the organism via a chemical or humoral messenger or some aspect of stimulation of the nervous system allowing it to mobilize and integrate its activities for reparative processes.

Man is unique in that he responds not only to actual danger but also to threats and symbols of danger. Indeed, such threats, or the anticipation of noxious stimuli, may elicit responses of far greater magnitude and duration than the actual injury itself. One can think of many examples of this: sitting in the dentist's waiting room or chair, a child anticipating a spanking, etc. Similarly, the protective adaptive reaction, when sustained, may itself be far more dangerous and damaging than the noxious agent *per se*. A rise in blood pressure in response to anger or fear may have some useful pupose in animals, but the irritable executive whose blood pressure boils over and who consequently has a stroke in response to some minor vexation is having an inappropriate adaptive response far more dangerous to his life than the original irritant. Quite probably, emotional stress in humans has more profound effects than physical stress, as demonstrated by the Harvard crewing studies. Emotional stress results in adaptive responses which might once have been useful in our evolutionary progenitors but which have now become injurious to us.

It is difficult in our present frame of reference to conceive of cancer as something that might once have been useful or reparative. The cancer patient today is generally avoided by family, friends, and even physicians, and the diagnosis is considered to be an ill omen and tantamount to a death sentence. Cancer conveys the fear of prolonged pain and suffering, loss of attractiveness and social esteem, or the contemplation of disfiguring surgery—as occurs in neck and head dissection or in a colostomy. The situation is most reminiscent of the Biblical leper who was analagously consumed by a process that was decaying or putrescent. Cancer may indeed be considered obscene in the original sense of that word as defined in the *Oxford English Dictionary:* "offensive to the senses or to taste or refinement; disgusting, repulsive, filthy, foul, abominable, loathsome." The distinguished psychiatrist Karl Menninger noted that "the very word 'cancer' is said to kill some patients who would not have succumbed (as rapidly) to the malignancy from which they suffer." The euphemism "moon children" has replaced "cancer" in astrological charts. Even a Federal Law—the 1966 Freedom of Information Act—singles out cancer as the only disease exempt from disclosure, since it would be an "unwarranted invasion of personal privacy."

The term "cancer" is Latin, derived from the Green *karkinos*, both meaning "crab," and according to Galen so called because the swollen veins surrounding the affected part resembled a crab's limbs. Many other interpretations relating to the crab have been assigned to cancer: for instance, its ability to move quickly and silently in all directions, or its similarity to the pincer-like action of the crab claw in eating away tissue; these, however, have no etymological basis. The dictionary defines it as "a malignant growth tumor in different parts of the body that tends to spread indefinitely and to *reproduce* itself as also to return after removal." The earliest English reference I can find is a quotation dating back to 1601: "Cancer is a swelling or sore comming of melancholy bloud, about which the veins appear of a blacke or swert colour spread in manner of a creifish clees [crayfish claws]." How appropriate that the adjective "melancholy" should have been used. The symbolic aspects of the term are deftly explored in Sontag's current best-seller, *Illness as Metaphor*.

Does any of this have any practical significance in terms of the prevention of cancer? I think so. It should be possible with the discoveries we have discussed and with further refinements in psychological testing to identify a population that is at greater risk for certain types of cancer—an identification facilitated by a knowledge of predisposing heredity and environmental factors. If hormonal and immunologic alterations play a role in the development and course of certain malignancies, it should be possible to pinpoint those changes and utilize them for predictive purposes; indeed, this is already being done in cancer of the breast and uterus. Similarly, if such factors play an active role in the development of the process, it may be possible to alter them artificially with beneficial consequences. The Nobel laureate Rosalyn Yalow recently noted that the pituitary hormone ACTH is found in virtually all primary lung carcinomas, irrespective of cell type. Perhaps determination of plasma ACTH may have a role in the clinical management of this disease. Parenthetically, what is the significance of this finding in the light of our knowledge of the importance of ACTH in the responses to stress and the growing evidence that stress may play a determinant role in the development of lung cancer in cigarette smokers? If depression plays a major role in the development of carcinoma, perhaps the development of objective chemical tests to identify such an emotional state could prove extremely useful.

More importantly, if stress or noxious influences can cause cancer, why cannot their antithesis have the opposite effect, as has been suggested for other diseases of adaptation? Adam Smith's *Powers of Mind* cites, for example, the interesting case of Norman Cousins, the distinguished editor of the *Saturday Review of Literature*, who was crippled with a severe and progressive form of arthritis. Having read Selye's work, Cousins reasoned that he could reverse the process by reversing noxious stimuli and apparently "laughed himself well." Several years ago, J. I. Rodale, the founder of *Prevention*, wrote a book entitled *Happy People Rarely Get Cancer*. Why is it that nuns, Mormons, Christian Scientists, and Seventh-Day Adventists have less cancer? Is it because they have found some inner peace or life style which insulates them from stress?

Finally, there is increasing evidence that the patient's emotional participation may play an important role in the course of his disease. This is emphasized in LeShan's book, *You Can Fight for Your Life*, and more recently by the Simontons, who are particularly interested in visual imagery and utilization of techniques such as biofeedback and hypnosis. In a recent publication, they report that during a four-year period, they treated 159 patients with "medically incurable" malignancies and average life expectancies of a year. They claim that of those who have died, the average survival time was over 20 months, and of the 63 surviving, 22% had "no evidence of disease" and tumors were regressing in 19%. Treatment centers utilizing the Simonton technique are now springing up all over the country. If such a biofeedback technique does have merit, then it can certainly be refined and improved.

Biofeedback has been demonstrated to be of significant value where the patient has an immediate opportunity to discern whether or not certain emotional states or thoughts are producing a desired effect. Thus, connected to an appropriate sensing and recording apparatus, the individual may determine whether thinking one way or another causes his blood pressure or pulse or skin temperature to rise, determinations he would not be able to make under normal circumstances in which there is no tangible evidence that the desired effect is being achieved. The situation is analogous to being placed in a car blindfolded on a racetrack and having to drive completely around the track without any interference. This would be an extremely difficult task; but if the driver had a set of earphones and received a signal in the left ear if he were getting too close to an impediment on the left, or a similar signal in the right ear if some danger were on the right, he could probably negotiate the course very satisfactorily. That is the type of assistance and reinforcement that biofeedback provides. With increasing use and experience, one could probably learn to circumnavigate the course at relatively high speeds.

It is known empirically that such emotional states as tranquility or relaxation are associated with a reduction in blood pressure. This provides a basis for using such techniques as transcendental meditation or the relaxation response to lower blood pressure. In this approach to cancer therapy, however, there would not appear to be the same degree of quantitative or qualitative effectiveness as formal biofeedback techniques provide. Mental imagery techniques and changing of the patient's attitude may very well be steps in the right direction, but what is needed is a more precise means of measuring whether or not the desired result is being accomplished. Otherwise, one is very much like the blindfolded racetrack driver.

There are certain nonspecific markers for malignancy such as the carcinoembryogenic assay, and other more specific indicators for certain types of cancer such as acid phosphatase for cancer of the prostate. No one knows exactly how rapidly these fluctuate with the state of the malignant process; but if it were possible to monitor the activity of malignancy by some such objective criterion, then the efficacy of such imagery or other biofeedback techniques would be greatly enhanced.

There are many claims for cancer cures, all with their zealous advocates: mineral waters, comfrey and other herbs, voodoo, yoga, faith healing, krebiozen, acupuncture, laetrile, and various shrines. It would seem unreasonable to state that there is not a scintilla of truth in any of these claims, and yet it is perfectly obvious that none of these agencies is consistently effective. What could they have in common?

The clue may be found in the case history cited by Klopfer in his description of a patient with a far advanced lymphosarcoma who begged to be treated with krebiozen. Following the initial administration of this substance, his tumor masses "melted like snowballs on a hot stove." Where previously he had required an oxygen mask to breathe, he was now able to fly a plane at 12,000 feet without any effort. However, after some unfavorable publicity appeared suggesting that krebiozen was ineffective, he again became bedridden. His physician, in desperation, then told him the reports were inaccurate and based upon deteriorated preparations of the drug, and that he would be given a stronger dose of a more active potent principle. Actually, he was given *distilled water*, but again the disease disappeared rapidly. When, however, it was announced that the Food and Drug Administration and the American Medical Association had found krebiozen to be worthless, he thereupon succumbed to his disease within a matter of days.

In a discussion in one of the papers presented at the New York Academy of Sciences International Conference on Immunology of Cancer, reference is made to the "Berkley-Smythe effect" noted at McMaster University in Toronto in a study utilizing BCG vaccine in patients with lung cancer. The initial program was undertaken by an enthusiastic thoracic surgeon given the pseudonym "Berkley-Smythe," who had a positive, personalized, optimistic approach and achieved rather remarkable results. Because of this, the study was, subsquently, greatly expanded but now carried out by different staff physicians. Surprisingly, absolutely no improvement was noted in the new group of patients. I should like to quote from the discussion:

> We then sat down and said, why is this? Why are we seeing no beneficial effect? Why did the first four patients do so much better? We said, let's try to visualize the patient who is in the cubicle when Berkley-Smythe walks in and says, "Good afternoon, Mr. Featherwick. It's good to see that you've recovered from your operation. You are feeling much better now, aren't you? Mr. Featherwick says, "Oh yes, I'm feeling a hell of a lot better than I did when I had my chest

tube in, and I really feel like I'm on the road to recovery." Berkley-Smythe then agrees that he's doing very well, indeed, but that his outlook might be even better with some additional treatment. "We now have a good way to treat you that we've learned about from experimental animal studies and from other people's work with patients who have a similar problem to yours. We would be glad to do this for you if you would like to try it; wouldn't you Featherwick? OK, just sign this consent form. You know it's a pretty benign treatment. There are some complications that could occur, but they aren't nearly as bad as the operation that you came through well." All of which is true. So the patient is entered into the study and comes back every visit to see Berkely-Smythe, who is smiling and enthusiastic, and the patient is smiling enthusiastically and doing well.

On the other hand, there are doctors in the immunotherapy clinic who don't have the aura of Berkley-Smythe. Dr. Marvin Milquetoast is one. Marvin goes to see a patient (let's call him Mr. Thanapolensis) whom he has never seen before and introduces himself as Marvin Milquetoast, the immunotherapist. "Your doctor," says Marvin, "has referred you here for our experimental treatment protocol. Now, we really don't have any idea whether this treatment is any good or not, but there isn't much else we can do for you, so we'd like to include you in this experiment. You may get the treatment or you may not, but if you'd like to join anyway and maybe get a chance at it, we'd be happy to have you. Before you sign, though, I have to tell you that you'll get sores on your arms and legs, you may get a fever or throw up, and you may get granulomatous hepatitis, or even anaphylaxis and die. But you'll probably be okay. Now you understand that, don't you?" So Mr. Thanapolensis signs up, and away we go. But somehow, Dr. Milquetoast's patients don't do very well.

We've all seen in one way or another this phenomenon, which I have termed the Berkley-Smythe effect, the powerful influence of psychologic suggestion. We have recently learned that it is sometimes possible to convince a patient to lower his own blood pressure. Maybe it is even possible that psychologic forces might help a patient to subdue his own tumor. We also see the Berkley-Smythe effect acting on ourselves and other investigators, and I think we must be very careful that it does not influence our objectivity, particularly as we report our results in meetings like this one.

Both of these anecdotes are strongly reminiscent of a well-recognized phenomenon in clinical medicine known as the "placebo" effect, which is generally acknowledged but poorly understood. It must in some way activate whatever self-regulatory mechanisms lie latent in the body as a factor in the expectation or hope of cure. It seems likely that such a compelling belief, hope, or trust is also the basis of those unusual instances of sudden remission from cancer for which there is no rational explanation. (I do not include vitamin C in the list of the above placebo-type "cures" because there is increasing evidence that this substance may play an important pharmacologic role in the therapeutic management of malignancies, and the profound effects of stress on vitamin C metabolism makes such a relationship plausible.)

The National Cancer Institute estimates that 80–90 percent of human cancers are attributable to environmental carcinogens; and this, of course, implies that cancer is largely preventable, and quite likely, a disease of man-made origin. *The New York Times* (June 17, 1978) quoted the Director of the National Cancer Institute as conceding that "a rosy view of the cancer problem is unwarranted." He suggested that more money ought to be spent on preventing cancer by changing the environment, and less on "unproven hypotheses" such as that cancer is caused by viruses. The next day's paper carried a page-one article indicating that spiritual healing was gaining ground among Catholics and Episcopalians, citing certain cancer patients "who recovered or enjoyed long remissions, or whose final days were painless."

I find an appealing link between these two items because they refer to both the external and internal environment and raise important questions. Hardly a week goes by that we do not find some report of epidemiologists studying an outbreak of cancer in a certain locality or among a specific group of individuals. Epidemiology attempts to deal with certain basic questions as to where a given disease is found, where it flourishes and when and where it is not found. Professor Danishevsky of Moscow divided epidemiologic climates into two categories: a so-called "macroclimate" which has to do with measurable factors such as temperature, humidity, atmospheric pressure, and air pollution, and a "microclimate" which represents the sum of the intimate sociologic, spiritual, and habitational conditions in which a given individual finds himself. As we shall see, there is a strong support for the position that cancer appears to be a disease of civilization and environment, and it may be more related to the "microclimate" than the "macroclimate."

The renowned medical missionary, Dr. Albert Schweitzer, wrote:

On my arrival in Gabon in 1913, I was astonished to encounter no cases of cancer. . . . I cannot, of course, say positively that there was no cancer at all; but, like other frontier doctors, I can only say that if any cases existed, they must have been quite rare. In the course of the years, we have seen cases of cancer in growing numbers in our region. My observations incline me to attribute this to the fact that the natives are living more and more after the manner of the whites. . . .

The celebrated anthropologist and Arctic explorer, Vilhjalmur Stefansson, in a book entitled *Cancer: Disease of Civilization?*, noted the absence of cancer in the Eskimos upon his initial arrival in the Arctic, but a subsequent increase in the incidence of the disease as closer contact with white civilization was established. He quotes Sir Robert McCarrison, a physician who surveyed 11,000 Hunza natives in Kashmir from 1904–1911, and concluded that cancer was unknown among them. In addition to their diet, the Hunzas were "far removed from the refinements of civilization. Certain of these races are of magnificent physique, preserving until late in life the character of youth; they are unusually fertile and long-lived and *endowed with nervous systems of notable stability.* . . ."

Dr. Morley Roberts' *Malignancy and Evolution* (1926) contained the observation: "I take the view commonly held that, whatever its origin, cancer is very largely a disease of civilization," and he was referring to a wide body of literature, such as Dr. Charles Powell's *The Pathology of Cancer* (1908) which stated: "There can be little doubt that the various influences grouped under the title of civilization play a part in producing a tendency to Cancer."

The earliest reference I have been able to find to support this thesis is LeConte's "Statistical Researches," in which he quotes the unpublished "Memoir on the Frequency of Cancer" which the French author Tanchou addressed to the French Academy of Science in 1843:

M. Tanchou is of the opinion that cancer, like insanity, increases in a direct ratio to the civilization of the country, and of the people. And it is certainly a remarkable circumstance, doubtless in no small degree flattering to the vanity of the French *savant*, that the average mortality rate from Cancer in Paris during 11 years is about 0.80 per 1000 living annually, while it is only 0.20 per 1000 in London! Estimating the intensity of civilization by these data, it clearly follows that Paris is four times more civilized than London!

In an article in the journal *Cancer,* in July 1927, Dr. William Howard Hay wrote:

> A study of the distribution of cancer, among the races of the entire earth, shows a cancer ratio in about proportion to which civilized living predominates; so evidently something inherent in the habits of civilization is responsible for the difference of cancer incidence as compared with the uncivilized races and tribes. Climate has nothing to do with this difference, as witness the fact that tribes living naturally will show a complete absence of cancer until mixture with more civilized man corrupts the naturalness of habit, and just as these habits conform to those of civilization, even so does cancer begin to show its head. . . .

One of the most impressive arguments is to be found in Dr. Alexander Berglas' work *Cancer: Its Nature, Cause and Cure,* published in Paris in 1957. Throughout this book runs the theme that cancer is a disease from which primitive peoples are relatively or wholly free. Berglas declares: ". . . there is as yet no remedy for cancer; it is not infectious, and it is the most frequent cause of death in highly developed countries (exclusive of death due to wear and old age); . . . everyone of us is threatened with death from cancer because of our *inability to adapt to present day living conditions.*" It is in his Preface, however, that I find the most significant, prophetic and useful commentary:

> Over the years, cancer research has become the domain of specialists in various fields. Despite the outstanding contributions of the scientists, we have been getting farther away from our goal, the curing of cancer. This specialized work, and the knowledge gained through the study of individual processes, had the peculiar result of becoming an obstacle to the study of the whole.
> More than thirty years in the field of cancer research have convinced me that it is not to our advantage to continue along this road of detailed analysis. I have come to the conclusion that cancer may perhaps be just another intelligible natural process whose cause is to be found in our environment and mode of life.

The current thrust of cancer research appears to be in the area of environmental carcinogens, especially those of dietary or atmospheric origin. In addition to such an epidemiologic approach, what is required is an endemiologic investigation, the search for common factors that lie *within* the affected population. What is needed is a new breed of physician, fluent not only in the technical and scientific advances that medicine has to offer in physiology, biochemistry, and psychology, but equipped with a sufficient background in literature, history, philosophy, and the humanities to enable him to evaluate the individual from a truly holistic viewpoint.

There is sometimes a tendency to minimize the significance of observations made by earlier investigators because they lack "scientific proof" or "statistical significance," but I have emphasized the opinions of 18th- and 19th-century physicians in this presentation since these doctors undoubtedly enjoyed a doctor–patient relationship that is not often seen today. By virtue of their own cultural background and their freedom to spend more time with their patients, their perception and appreciation of the significance of developmental and personal environmental factors were indubitably enhanced. Indeed, "it is sometimes much more important to know what kind of patient has the disease than what kind of disease the patient has."

Louis Pasteur, who was preoccupied with microbes as a cause of disease, had many debates with his contemporary, Claude Bernard, who, as we have seen, stressed the importance of the body's own equilibrium and the significance of the *milieu intérieur* or internal environment. It is reported that on his deathbed Pasteur said: "*Bernard avait raison. Le germe n'est rien, c'est le terrain qui est tout.*" [Bernard was right. The microbe is nothing, the soil is everything.] In other words, the type of patient may be more important than the nature of the disease in determining the outcome.

Sir William Osler, possibly the greatest of all clinicians, used to tell his students: "Show me what goes on in a man's head, and I will tell you what will become of his tuberculosis," and that was long before we knew anything about a drug called cortisone, which promotes the rapid spread of tuberculosis, or before we had discovered that hormones such as this were the hallmark of the response to stress. Significantly enough, he also observed that faith was the physician's greatest aid.

The causal relationship between stress and numerous disorders has been increasingly accepted since Selye's revolutionary concept of "diseases of adaptation." There is no longer any doubt that stress can influence all human disease. Its relationship to cancer may be difficult to "prove" to a statistician's satisfaction, for reasons noted above, but that does not exclude the possibility or likelihood that it will soon join the ranks of what might be more appropriately relabeled "diseases of maladaptation."

References

Cannon, W. B. *The Wisdom of the Body.* New York: W. W. Norton, 1932.

Dubos, R. Homeostasis, illness and biological creativity. *Lahey Clinic Foundation Bulletin*23:94–100, 1974.

Dubos, R. *Man Adapting.* New Haven: Yale University Press, 1965.

Dunbar, F. *Emotions and Bodily Changes.* New York: Columbia University Press, 1954.

Dunbar, F., and Rosch, P. J. Illness syndromes: High disability. In *Psychiatry in the Medical Specialties.* New York: McGraw-Hill, 1959, pp. 155–317.

Fox, B. H. Premorbid psychological factors as related to cancer incidence. *J. Behav. Med.*1:45–133, 1978.

Holmes, T. H., and Rahe, R. H. The social readjustment rating scale. *J. Psychosom. Med.*11:213–218, 1967.

LeShan, L. *You Can Fight for Your Life.* New York: M. Evans, 1977.

Mason, J. W. Psychologic stress and endocrine function. In Sachar, F. J. (Ed.), *Topics in Psychoendocrinology.* New York: Grune & Stratton, 1965.

Mason, J. W. Specificity in the organization of neuroendocrine profiles. In *Frontiers of Neurology and Neuroscience Research.* Toronto: Neuroscience Institute, 1974, pp. 68–80.

Rosch, P. J. Stress: Its relationship with illness. In *Traumatic Medicine and Surgery for the Attorney.* London: Butterworths, 1960, pp. 261–364.

Rosch, P. J. Growth and development of the stress concept and its significance in clinical medicine. In *Modern Trends in Endocrinology.* New York: Paul B Hoeber; London: Butterworths, 1958, pp. 278–297.

Selye, H. *Stress in Health and Disease.* London: Butterworths, 1976.

Selye, H. *Stress without Distress.* Philadelphia: J. B. Lippincott, 1974.

Selye, H. *The Stress of Life.* New York: McGraw-Hill, 1956.

Selye, H. *Stress.* Montreal: Acta, 1950.

Selye, H., and Rosch, P. J. The renaissance in endocrinology. In *Medicine and Science.* New York: International University Press, 1954, pp. 30–49.

Selye, H., and Rosch, P. J. Integration of endocrinology. In *Glandular Physiology and Therapy.* Philadelphia: J. B. Lippincott Co., 1954, pp. 1–100.

Simonton, B. C., Mathews-Simonton, S., and Creighton, J. *Getting Well Again.* Los Angeles: J. P. Tacher, 1978.

Sontag, S. *Illness as Metaphor.* New York: Farrar, Straus, and Giroux, 1977.

Stefansson, V. *Cancer: Disease of Civilization?* New York: Hill and Wang, 1960.

Thomas, C. B. *Habits of Nervous Tension: Clues to the Human Condition.* 725 Wolfe Street, Baltimore, Maryland 21205, 1977.

Thomas, C. B., and Greenstreet, R. L. Psychological characteristics in youth as predictors of five disease states: Suicide, mental illness, hypertension, coronary heart disease, and tumor. *Johns Hopkins Med. J.*132:16–43, 1973.

18

Death Not the Mysterium Tremendum: A Summary Overview

Stacey B. Day, M.D., Ph.D., D.Sc.

It would need one of exceptional wisdom to reach a simple conclusion in summing up the many thoughtful interdisciplinary perspectives discussed in this book on *Cancer, Stress, and Death*. None would disagree that *death* is the great separator. The husband is forever parted from his wife, the father from the son, the mother from the child, the neighbor from the community. This separation may occur in isolation or as an element of death *en masse*. In our times, and in our days, we live under conditions in which virtually entire nations, entire societies, entire cities, may be suddenly destroyed. Death has many meanings, and they change with culture and society. And with this change has come a certain blunting of the once-held awe of death, a blunting of the supreme *mysterium tremendum*.

Today we are able to discuss death from every possible viewpoint, physiological, neuroendocrinological, social, behavioral, and as a dynamic of cultural anthropology. Where fear of death

Stacey B. Day • Member and Professor, Sloan-Kettering Institute for Cancer Research, New York, New York 10021.

exists, it is, as often as not, *fear in anticipation* of death, rather than fear of the event itself. This is especially so in cancer patients. It is as much to what goes before, the aura, the crisis (real or imaginary), the fear of the end being ultimately at hand, as to the final act that the apparatus of ministration and help has to address itself. *How* we provide help, and in what sense we view each unique death, of others as eventually our own, will depend to a considerable degree on how we, as a society, have handled the cultural transformations of our times, providing wisdom for our fellows as much as for ourselves. Cancer and death are entering more and more into the public consciousness, and, in proportion to the stress caused by this encumbrance, society is increasingly ready to discuss and endeavor to understand this human situation. There *is* a willingness to work toward mitigating the fear, the hurt, and the pain that characterize the stress of cancer in relation to death and dying. Traditionally in Christian society there have been psychological barriers to frankness in facing both cancer and death. In Ireland and France the "conspiracy of silence" is still the accepted way of facing cancer and death. Any physician who has practiced or spent time in these countries will know at first hand the extraordinary burden of stress that accompanies a cancer death, not only for the patient, who ostensibly does not know that he is facing death, but for the family, which *does* know but by custom and culture may not tell the patient. Families may be divided; financial burdens may become intolerable; and even long after the death, hostility toward various parties, including the physician, may remain.

Many of these attitudes and the problems they engender have been discussed in the accounts presented in this book.

In virtually all areas of our cultural transformation, there is a need for a general reeducation toward an appreciation of our living and the content of human life. With respect to cancer, the papers in this volume discuss many attitudes, including the abiding reluctance of many to accept a patient-as-a-person concept. Many physicians still concentrate upon the disease, upon cancer as an organ diathesis, almost to the exclusion of consideration of the patient himself! As a result, severe stress is not uncommonly found to be exerted all around: upon the patient, upon the physician, upon the general nursing and paramedical staff, upon the family, and upon society.

All of us create our own attitudes and our own prejudices. Most of us are fond of these creations, which can with paradoxical ease see death as a tragic parting and, almost simultaneously, view it quite dispassionately, with a detached composure. Consider the following comment that "Death Makes our Vacancies" from *The New York Times* (February 26, 1978).

> *"Awaiting Orders.* When old soldiers die, the Army takes care of their wives... Last week, the wife of... was accepted for residence at a home for Army widows in Washington... There is a waiting list, though, and Mrs.... will wait her turn for a one bedroom apartment with kitchen, bath and dining area. How long a wait, no one can say. 'Death makes our vacancies,' said the home's administrative officer."

Whatever is believed about death in general—that it is the great leveler, the great equalizer, that the heroes' death of *The Charge of the Light Brigade* is more noble than 200 persons dying in an airplane disaster or 10,000 dying in an earthquake or cyclone—in terms of *cancer and death,* as the accounts here testify, the most desolating breakdowns leading to stress are breaches in communication between the patient, the physician, and the family. Cultural sharing and harmonious attitudes, as well as awareness, suggest that *real* educational understanding can be achieved. But such understanding must be reached in good faith within the broad fellowship of society. No matter how much a small group may deliberate or plan in good faith, it will become nothing but a clan or cult of devotees with pedagogic interests and dedication unless a firm societal, holistic, mutually shared, open empathy of mind can be established with all in society. This should be the aim of the self-education process, some background points of which are commented on here.

Shading Responses

I have often wondered why men hang on to life as if it were personal property—much as they might hang on to a suit or a pair of trousers. Possibly rationalizing a little too simply, for myself as a physician, I am one with old Dr. Parr who sighed in his last illness,

"Oh, if I can only live till strawberries come!" John Burroughs said the old scholar imagined that if he could weather it till then, the berries would carry him through. "No doubt he has turned from the drugs and nostrums, or from the hateful food, to the memory of the pungent, penetrating, and unspeakably fresh quality of the strawberry with the deepest longing." If a full life can end with a strawberry death, embodying as it were the first glow and ardor of young summer, then I think life will have unsheathed its taste and rewarded the appetite of any man. But to hang on to life as if it were a personal possession seems, to me at least, to invite great stress.

The intellectually and educationally superior individual is no doubt capable of handling anxiety and stress more effectively than most people, but even *he* may be susceptible to intense and debilitating fears. Uncertainty and the fear of failure in cancer therapy are essential features of anxiety for most patients. The superior individual may surpass others in raising questions, foreseeing complications, and discovering sources of possible failure, by virtue of his potential assets, but there is no certainty that even he will more easily face ideas of mourning or of death with equanimity.

Anxiety may be defined as "a specific conscious inner attitude and a peculiar-feeling state characterized by a number of vectors." These vectors include:

(1) A physically and a mentally painful awareness of being powerless to do anything about a personal matter
(2) Premonition of an impending and almost inevitable danger
(3) A tense and physically exhausting alertness as if facing an emergency
(4) An apprehensive self-absorption which interferes with an effective and advantageous solution of reality problems
(5) An irresolvable doubt concerning the nature of the threatening cancer

Generally speaking, the more passive the individual's behavior, the more strongly stressed his attitude of passive acceptance is likely to be.

Practically every human being experiences anxiety states of varying intensity at one time or another. Awareness of one's powerlessness causes apprehension because of its association with a dread of failure. This dread is due in large measure to ignorance as to what one actually fears. Among the Eskimo Innuit of Alaska north of the Brooks Range, I have rarely found any dread or fear of putting to sea in the Arctic Ocean—ice-bound and hostile to an alien visitor. What was for me a situation of absolute powerlessness was for them a commonplace occurrence. And even dreaded danger was for them not necessarily equated with death, I found. These values are culture-oriented. Physical injury, social status, reduction of value, may represent impending danger, and these may all be very real fears in patients hospitalized with cancer.

To the psychoanalyst, sexual drive with its gratifications is the most fundamental motivation of human behavior. Observations from World War II—in the concentration camps—and my observations among the Innuit Eskimos (who know little if anything at all of "cancer"), suggest that sex is *not* the most basic drive. *Physical survival* is the most basic. These perspectives must be kept in mind as stress-provocative agents in the cancer patient to whom both sex and survival may be important basic drives. Similarly, such issues as fitness and effectiveness, adaptation, biological clocks—the physiologic process of time—use by the patient, competition, the parliament of genes, and the characteristics of a given patient as determined by his genes, all combine to arrange variations on which the ultimate life–death play is acted out. Handling these biologic and physiologic imperatives by cultural strategies has a critical part in the support or in the eventual failure of the "forces" that support the body. Many strategies directed to this aspect of dissolution of the patient have been presented in reasonable perspective in the text.

In all these physical phenomena, there are usually concordant mental phenomena—the possibility that mental states are identical with certain physical processes such as brain processes. Professor Wolfgang Luthe wrote in his chapter of some of these aspects of cancer, stress, and death.

There is no single resolution, no one answer. There is, I feel, only a certain harmony. If one has stood high atop the Himalayas, and looked down into the valleys, many miles or more deep, one senses a strange combination of limits—depths and heights relating to each other in harmony. So should life and death blend into a holistic understanding. The physician, as much as any other person, should recognize a patient with cancer as a person. Even though the patient is ill, he himself still has an idea of personality. He sees himself as an individual still playing out an important role in life—his death. Everything in a physician's training *should* have moved him toward the recognition of the patient's individuality, of his being a person—an extraordinary composite of body and mind, sensitivity and character, a look, a turn, a touch, a hand on the shoulder, a smile, wind in the hair on a warm summer day.

Nor should the physician, in my view, equate everything in "numbers of days." The dialectic of experience is in time. Time begins to exist with man through and in his self-awareness. In enhancing this, the cancer physician passes immeasurably beyond minutes, hours, days, in his relationship with his patient.

Si vis vitam, para mortem. The dying still share life with the living. Life becomes endurable for the cancer patient, less burdened with stress, when all those about him—especially in the face of death—encourage him to grow, to give further truthfulness to his life, and to share his unique personal, psychological and cultural *allness,* his *oneness,* with all who come into contact with him in his illness—with his physician, the general staff, his family, and society as a whole. The sharing process, in my view, does not cease until separation, or death, is complete.

Recommended Reading

Aldrich, C. K. Personality factors and mortality in the relocation of the aged. *Gerontologist* 4:92–93, 1964.

Ammon, G., and Hameister, H. J.: Tod und Sterben als Identitätsproblem: ich psychologische und gruppendynamische Aspekte. [Ego psychological and group dynamic aspects of death and dying.] *Dynam. Psychiat. (Berlin)* 8:129–142, 1975.

Arce, L. Somatopsychic disease. *Psychosomatics* 13:191–196, 1972.

Bacon, G. E., George, R., Koeff, S. T., and Howatt, W. F. Plasma corticoids in the respiratory distress syndrome and in normal infants. *Pediatrics* 55:500–502, 1975.

Barnes, B. O., Ratzenhofer, M., and Gisi, R. The role of natural consequences in the changing death patterns. *J. Amer. Geriat. Soc.* 22:176–179, 1974.

Bartko, J. J., and Patterson, R. D. Survival among healthy old men: A multivariate analysis. In: Granick, S., and Patterson, R. D. (Eds.), *Human Aging II. An Eleven-year Follow-up Biomedical and Behavioral Study.* Washington, D.C.: U.S. Department of Health, Education, and Welfare, 1971, pp. 105–117.

Bowers, M. K., Jackson, E. N., Knight, J. A., and LeShan, L. *Counseling the Dying.* London, New York, Toronto: Thomas Nelson and Sons, 1964, p. 183.

Bugen, L. A. Human grief: A model for prediction and intervention. *Am. J. Orthopsychiatry* 47:196–206, 1977.

Bührmann, M. V. The dying child. *S. Afr. Med. J.* 47:1114–1116, 1973.

Cameron, J. M., and Watson, E. Sudden death in infancy in Inner North London. *J. Path.* 116:55–61, 1975.

Carey, A. Helping the child and the family cope with death. *Int. J. Fam. Counsel.* 5:58–63, 1977.

Clayton, P. J., Halikas, J. A., Maurice, W. L., and Robins, E. Anticipatory grief and widowhood. *Br. J. Psychiatry* 122:47–51, 1973.

Coolidge, J. C. Unexpected death in a patient who wished to die. *J. Amer. Psychoanal. Ass.* 17:413–420, 1969.

Day, Stacey B. *Death and Attitudes towards Death.* Minneapolis: Bell Museum of Pathobiology, University of Minnesota Medical School, 1972.

Day, Stacey B. *Tuluak and Amaulik. Dialogues on Death and Mourning with the Innuit Eskimo of Point Barrow and Wainwright, Alaska.* Minneapolis: Bell Museum of Pathobiology, University of Minnesota Medical School, 1973.

Dimsdale, J. E. Emotional causes of sudden death. *Am. J. Psychiatry* 134:1361–1366, 1977.

Dubovsky, S. L., Getto, C. J., Gross, S. A., and Paley, J. A. Impact on nursing care and mortality: Psychiatrists on the coronary care unit. *Psychosomatics* 18(3):18–27, 1977.

Duhl, L. J. A memorial to Erich Lindemann. *J. Commun. Psychol.* 3:300–302, 1975.

Eckert, E. E. Plötzlicher und unerwarteter Tod im Kleinkindesalter und elektromagnetisch Felder. [Sudden, unexpected death of infants and electromagnetic fields.] *Med. Klin.* 71:1500–1505, 1976.

Eliot, R. S. Emotional stress and coronary artery disease. *J. S. C. Med. Ass.* Supp. 72:88–95, 1976.

Eliot, R. S., Clayton, F. C., Pieper, G. M., and Todd, G. L. Influence of environmental stress on pathogenesis of sudden cardiac death. *Fed. Proc.* 36:1719–1724, 1977.

Escoffier-Lanbiotte. Le medecin devant la mort. II. L'aide aux moribonds. *Bruxelles-Med.* 57:475–478, 1977.

Eyer, J. Does unemployment cause the death rate peak in each business cycle? A multifactor model of death rate change. *Int. J. Health Serv.* 7:625–662, 1977.

Fredrick, J. F. Grief as a disease process. *Omega (Westport, Conn.)* 7:297–305, 1977.

Goldberg, E. L., and Comstock, G. W. Life events and subsequent illness. *Am. J. Epidemiol.* 104:146–158, 1976.

Goldfarb, A. I., Shahinian, S. P., and Burr, H. T. Death rate of relocated nursing home residents. In: Kent, D. P., Kastenbaum, R., and Sherwood, S. (Eds.), *Research Planning and Action for the Elderly: The Power and Potential of Social Science.* New York: Behavioral Publ., 1972, pp. 525–537.

Goldsmith, C. E. A theoretical analysis of attitudes of older people toward dying (Abstr.). *Diss. Abstr. Int.* B30:2401–B, 1969.

Goodfriend, M., and Wolpert, E. A. Death from fright: Report of a case and literature review. *Psychosom. Med.* 38:348–356, 1976.

Gow, C. M., and Williams, J. I. Nurses' attitudes toward death and dying: A causal interpretation. *Soc. Sci. Med.* 11:191–198, 1977.

Greene, W. A., Goldstein, S., and Moss, A. J. Psychosocial aspects of sudden death. A preliminary report. *A. M. A. Arch. Intern. Med.* 129:725–731, 1972.

Hackett, T. P., and Weisman, A. D. Reactions to the imminence of death. In: Gross, G. H., Wechsler, H., and Greenblat, M. (Eds.), *The Threat of Impending Disaster. Contributions to the Psychology of Stress.* Cambridge, Mass.: M.I.T. Press, 1964, pp. 300–311.

Haider, I. Attitudes toward death of psychiatric patients. *Int. J. Neuropsychiatry* 3: 10–14, 1967.

Harvey, W. P., and Levine, S. A. Paroxysmal ventricular tachycardia due to emotion. Possible mechanism of death from fright. *J.A.M.A.* 150:479–480, 1952.

Haynes, S. G., McMichael, A. J., and Tyroler, H. A. The relationship of normal, involuntary retirement to early mortality among U.S. rubber workers. *Soc. Sci. Med.* 11:105–114, 1977.

Hinton, J. M. The physical and mental distress of the dying. *Quart. J. Med.* 32:1–21, 1963.

Hinton, J. M. Distress in dying. In: Agate, J. N. (Ed.), *Medicine in Old Age.* Philadelphia: J. B. Lippincott, 1966, pp. 180–187.

Hinton, J. M. *Dying*. Second Edition. Baltimore: Penguin Books, 1972, p. 220.

Janssen, W. Todesfälle im Rahmen emotionaler Belastung. [Death within the framework of emotional stress.] *Beitr. Gerichtl. Med.* 33:97–102, 1975.

Jeffers, F. C., Nichols, C. R., and Eisdorfer, C. Attitudes of older persons toward death: A preliminary study. In: Tibbitts, C., and Donahue, W. (Eds.), *Social and Psychological Aspects of Aging*, Vol. I. New York and London: Columbia University Press, 1962, pp. 709–715.

Jeffers, F. C., and Verwoerdt, A. How the old face death. In: Busse, E. W., and Pfeiffer, E., (Eds.), *Behavior and adaptation in Late Life*. Boston: Little, Brown and Co., 1969, pp. 163–181.

Jennings, P. B. Adrenal cortical function at death as measured by level of circulating eosinophils. *Br. Med. J.* May 17: 1055–1058, 1952.

Kalish, R. A. Of social values and the dying: A defense of disengagement. *Fam. Coordin.* 21:81–94, 1972.

Kastenbaum, R.: The mental life of dying geriatric patients. *Gerontologist* 7:97–100, 1967.

Kimsey, L. R., Roberts, J. L., and Logan, D. L. Death, dying, and denial in the aged. *Am. J. Psychiatry* 129:161–166, 1972.

Kleiman, M. A., Mantell, J. E., and Alexander, E. S. Rx for social death: The cancer patient as counselor. *Community Ment. Health J.* 13:115–124, 1977.

Koskenvuo, K. Sudden deaths among Finnish conscripts. *Br. Med. J.* Dec. 11:1413–1415, 1976.

Kruck, F., Levi L., Eiff, A. W. von, Bohus, B., Kovách, A. G. B., Schaefer, H., Hippius, H., Andreani, D., Görres, A., and Richter-Heinrich, E. Diskussion. In: Eiff, A. W. von. (Ed.), *Seelische und körperliche Störungen durch Stress*. [Psychic and physical disturbances caused by stress.] Stuttgart: Gustav Fischer Verlag, 1976, pp. 218–233.

Kübler-Ross, E. The care of the dying. Whose job is it? *Psychiat. Med.* 1:103–107, 1970.

Kübler-Ross, E. Dying with dignity. *Canad. Nurse* 67:31–35, 1971.

Kübler-Ross, E. Death, the final stage of growth. Scarborough, England: Prentice Hall, 1975, p. 167.

Kübler-Ross, E. Image of growth and death. Scarborough, England: Prentice Hall, 1976, pp. 1–167.

Kübler-Ross, E. Death and dying. Toronto: Macmillan, 1970, p. 277.

Kübler-Ross, E. Wessler, S., and Avioli, L. V. On death and dying. *J.A.M.A.* 221: 174–179, 1972.

Lamerton, R. Distress of dying. *Brit. Med. J.* Aug. 5:351, 1972.

LeShan, L. Psychological states as factors in the development of malignant disease: A critical review. *J. Nat. Cancer Inst.* 22:1–18, 1959.

Manoach, M., Netz, H., Kariv, N., Kauli, N., and Gitter, S. Transient disturbances in atrioventricular conduction induced by restrained stress. *Adv. Cardiol.* 19:48–51, 1977.

McWeeny, P. M., and Emery, J. L. Unexpected postneonatal deaths (cot deaths) due to recognizable disease. *Arch. Dis. Childh.* 50:191–196, 1975.

Meyer, J. E. Psychoneuroses and neurotic reactions in old age. *J. Amer. Geriat. Soc.* 22:254–257, 1974.

Millerd, E. J. Health professionals as survivors. *J. Psychiat. Nurs.* 15(4):33–37, 1977.

Moos, R. H. Developmental life transitions: Deaht and bereavement. In: Moos, R. H. (Ed.), *Human Adaptation: Coping with Life Crises.* Lexington, Mass., Toronto, and London: D. C. Heath and Co., 1976, pp. 257–260.

Myler, B. B. Depression and death in the aged. (Abstr.). *Diss. Abstr. Int.* B28:2146–B, 1967.

Neels, R. J. The experience of dying and death. *N.Z. Med. J.*83:233–236, 1976.

Noyes, R., Jr. The dying patient: Establish his role to improve care. *Psychosomatics* 18(3):42–46, 1977.

Patterson, R. D., Freeman, L. C., and Butler, R. N. Psychiatric aspects of adaptation, survival, and death. In: Granick, S., and Patterson, R. D. (Eds.), *Human aging II. An Eleven-year Follow-up Biomedical and Behavioral Study.* Washington, D.C.: U.S. Department of Health, Education, and Welfare, 1971, pp. 63–94.

Paul, O., and Schatz, M. On sudden death. *Circulation*43:7–10, 1971.

Price, T. R., and Bergen, B. J. The relationship to death as a source of stress for nurses on a coronary care unit. *Omega (Westport, Conn.)*8:229–238, 1977.

Quint, J. C., and Strauss, A. L. Nursing students, assignments, and dying patients. A sociological approach concerning the problems of nursing faculty and students with the dying patient and death. *Nurs. Outlook*12:24–27, 1964.

Rahe, R. H., Bennett, L., Romo, M., Siltanen, P., and Arthur, R. J. Subjects' recent life changes and coronary heart disease in Finland. *Am. J. Psychiatry*130: 1973, 1222–1226.

Rosin, A. J., Assael, M., and Wallach, L. The influence of emotional reaction on the course of fatal illness. *Geriatrics*31:87–90, 1976.

Rowland, K. F. Environmental events predicting death for the elderly. *Psychol. Bull.*84:349–372, 1977.

Sauer, H. I. Migration and the risk of dying. *Proc. Soc. Statist. Sect., Am. Statist. Ass., Washington 1967* 1968, pp. 399–407.

Saunders, C. Care of the dying—5. Mental distress in the dying. *Nurs. Times*72: 1172–1174, 1976.

Schmale, A. H., Jr. Psychic trauma during bereavement. *Int. Psychiat. Clin*8:147–168, 1971.

Schwartz, A. M., and Karasu, T. B. Psychotherapy with the dying patient. *Am. J. Psychother.*31:19–35, 1977.

Simmons, L. W. The relation between the decline of anxiety-inducing and anxiety-resolving factors in a deteriorating culture and its relevance to bodily disease. In: Wolff, H. G., Wolf, S. G., Jr., and Hare, C. C. (Eds.), *Life Stress and Bodily Disease.* Baltimore: Williams and Wilkins Co., 1950, pp. 127–136.

Solnit, A. J., and Green, M. The pediatric management of the dying child. Part II. The child's reaction to the fear of dying. In: Solnit, A. J., and Provence, S. A. (Eds.), *Modern Perspectives in Child Development.* New York: International Universities Press, 1963, pp. 217–228.

Spiegel, J. P. Cultural variations in attitudes toward death and disease. In: Grosser, G. H., and Wechsler, H. (Eds.), *The Threat of Impending Disaster. Contributions to the Psychology of Stress.* Cambridge, Mass.: M.I.T. Press, 1964, pp. 283–299.

Spilka, B., Loeb, N., Weldon, L., Marker, T., and Albi, L. Those who are about to fly: Death concern and feelings and behavior about air travel. *Omega (Westport, Conn.)*8:107–116, 1978.

Squire, M. B. Death, dying and hard time therapy. *Int. J. Soc. Psychiatry*23:5–7, 1977.

Stubblefield, K. S. A preventive program for bereaved families. *Soc. Work Health Care*2:372–389, 1977.

Swenson, W. M. Attitudes toward death in an aged population. In: Tibbitts, C., and Donahue, W. (Eds.), *Social and Psychological Aspects of Aging*, Vol. I. New York and London: Columbia University Press, 1962, pp. 701–708.

Thomas, L. Notes of a biology-watcher. Facts of life. *New Eng. J. Med.*296:1462–1464, 1977.

Tietz, W., McSherry, L., and Britt, B. Family sequelae after a child's death due to cancer. *Am. J. Psychother.*31:417–425, 1977.

Vachon, M. L. S., Freedman, K., Formo, A., Rogers, J., Lyall, W. A. L., and Freeman, J. J. The final illness in cancer: The widow's perspective. *Canad. Med. Ass. J.*117:1151–1154, 1977.

Verwoerdt, A., and Elmore, J. L. Psychological reactions in fatal illness. I. The prospect of impending death. *J. Amer. Geriat. Soc.*15:9–19, 1967.

Walker, J. V. Attitudes to death. *Geront. Clin. (Basel)*10:304–308, 1968.

Weisman, A. D. *On Dying and Denying. A Psychiatric Study of Terminality*. New York: Behavioral Publ. 1972, p. 247.

Weisman, A. D. Coping with untimely death. In: Moos, R. H. (Ed.), *Human Adaptation: Coping with Life Crises*. Lexington, Mass., Toronto, and London: D. C. Heath and Co., 1976, pp. 261–274.

Wenkart, A. Death in life. *J. Existent.*8:75–90, 1967.

West, N. D. The psychology of death in geriatrics. *J. Amer. Geriat. Soc.*20:340–342, 1972.

Wolf, S. Psychosocial forces in myocardial infarction and sudden death. In: Levi, L. (Ed.), *Society, Stress, and Disease. 1. The Psychosocial Environment and Psychosomatic Diseases*. London, New York, Toronto: Oxford University Press, 1971, pp. 324–330.

Young, P. J. W. Scared to death. *Brit. Med. J.* Sept. 18:701, 1965.

Index